D1409270

PHARMACY TECHNICIAN
CAREER STARTER

PHARMACY TECHNICIAN
career starter

Felice Primeau Devine

New York

Copyright © 2002 LearningExpress, LLC.

All rights reserved under International and Pan-American Copyright Conventions.
Published in the United States by LearningExpress, LLC, New York.

Library of Congress Cataloging-in-Publication Data is available.

Printed in the United States of America
9 8 7 6 5 4 3 2 1
First Edition

ISBN 1-57685-410-8

For more information or to place an order, contact LearningExpress at:
    900 Broadway
    Suite 604
    New York, NY 10003

Or visit us at:
    www.learnatest.com

About the Author

Felice Primeau Devine is a writer from Albany, New York. She has worked in publishing for more than ten years as an editor, publicist, and brand director. She is the author of *U.S. Citizenship: A Step-by-Step Guide*, and coauthor of *Cosmetology Career Starter*.

Contents

Contents

Introduction

Why Become a Pharmacy Technician?

Pharmacy technicians, increasingly important members of the healthcare industry, work under the direct supervision of registered pharmacists. They assist pharmacists in their duties and their tasks may include serving patients, maintaining medication inventory, billing and crediting patients, preparing sterile products, maintaining patient records, compounding medications, and interpreting prescription orders.

One of the most basic reasons people become pharmacy technicians is interest in pharmacology. Indeed, pharmacology is a fascinating and constantly evolving field. You can rarely open a newspaper without finding an article about a new drug, a recalled drug, or a newly approved use for an existing drug.

Within this exciting field, employment opportunities for pharmacy technicians are excellent. Across the United States, people are living longer. As the population ages, the need for prescription medication increases. Along with that comes the increasing need for professionals to service the population and their prescription drugs—both pharmacists and pharmacy technicians. At the same time, as insurers, pharmacies, and healthcare providers continue to emphasize cost containment, the need for skilled pharmacy technicians grows. In fact, job demand for pharmacy technicians is projected to remain strong through the foreseeable future. The most recent *Occupational Outlook Handbook* published by the U.S. Department of Labor states that employment for pharmacy technicians will grow 10–20% from 1998–2008.

In addition to a positive employment outlook, pharmacy technicians have the opportunity to develop skills that can parlay into future careers. Certainly, if you start out as a pharmacy technician, you may one day wish to pursue a career as a registered pharmacist. If this is the case, you will have a strong foundation in pharmacology before you even set out on that journey.

Throughout this book, you will find information on what pharmacy technicians do on a day-to-day basis. You may already have a basic understanding of what it means to be a pharmacy technician—you did pick up this book, after all. This book will provide you with a more robust understanding of the field and how you should prepare for your first job—through training programs, certification, and the all-important job search. After digesting this information, you will be in a position to determine whether or not a career as a pharmacy technician is right for you. As you begin, it is important to recognize that there are a few key traits that are important for pharmacy technicians to possess. Typically people who enter the field:

▶ have strong communication and customer service skills
▶ can respect the confidentiality of patient information
▶ pay very close attention to detail
▶ possess a pleasant yet professional demeanor
▶ understand basic computer technology and can type accurately
▶ have an aptitude for mathematics

You will learn more about what it takes to succeed as a pharmacy technician in Chapter 6.

It's In the Details

It is crucial that prospective pharmacy technicians have the ability to do precise work—and enjoy it. When preparing prescriptions, missed details can mean the difference between life and death. The pharmacist with whom you work will check the prescriptions you fill, but as a skilled pharmacy technician, you should be able to do the work accurately on your own.

Once you've learned what it means to be a pharmacy technician from Chapter 1, you will find in Chapter 2 an extensive analysis of how to get the training you need. There are many training programs for pharmacy technicians in the United States, and by reading this book you will find out how to find the right program for you. For information on paying for your training, scholarships, grants, loans, and everything you need to know about how to find and apply for financial aid, turn to Chapter 3. This book will also explain what's required to become a certified pharmacy technician, including the exam, and why being able to use the designation of CPhT (or Certified Pharmacy Technician) is only one element that will determine the success and direction of your career. Recertification, required every two years if you are to continue to be a certified pharmacy technician, is also discussed.

After you complete your training, you will be eager to start working. Chapters 4 and 5 will show you how to conduct a job search and improve your job search skills. Then you will move on to Chapter 6, which is full of success strategies to help you make the most out of your first job and your career.

Where the Jobs Are

70% of pharmacy technicians work in retail pharmacies (both independently owned and those that are part of a chain). 20% work in hospital pharmacies and the remaining 10% of pharmacy technicians work in mail order pharmacies, clinics, pharmaceutical wholesalers, and for the government.

Source: U.S. Department of Labor

Interviews with pharmacy technicians who developed their careers in diverse ways appear throughout the book, providing you with valuable advice on what it takes to succeed. These professionals share their own experiences and discuss changes and critical issues in pharmacy practice— especially those that relate directly to the role of the pharmacy technician. The appendices at the back of the book not only list the most important organizations in the field but also point you toward helpful resources (books, websites, magazines, and journals).

To get the most out of this book, take a moment to look at what you will find in each chapter:

Chapter	Description
One The Hottest Careers for Pharmacy Technicians	This chapter will help you decide if a career as a pharmacy technician is right for you. It describes where the jobs are, and provides an overview of typical job responsibilities. It also contains salary surveys and other industry statistics.
Two All about Pharmacy Technician Education Programs	This chapter will help you decide which type of training program is most appropriate for your needs and plans. It describes a variety of types of training programs and provides sample course descriptions. Information on the pharmacy technician certification exam, is included.
Three Financial Aid: Discovering the Possibilities	Once you have decided what type of training is for you, this chapter will provide you with more information about schools that offer pharmacy technician programs. It also contains all the information you need to know about securing financial aid for the training program of your choice.
Four How to Land Your First Job: Networking, Conducting Your Job Search	This chapter explains how to find a job after you complete your training. It will help you learn how to conduct your job search through networking, research, industry publications, classified ads, online resources, visiting job fairs, and contacting job hotlines.
Five Resumes, Cover Letters, and the Job Interview Process	Chapter 5 will show you how to create an effective resume and cover letter. It tells you the most important items to include—and to avoid including—on your resume. You will discover how to complement a professional resume with a well-written cover letter, and what prospective employers look for during interviews. Sample interview questions are provided so you will have an idea of what you may be asked. Sample questions for you to ask of your interviewer are also provided.
Six How to Succeed Once You've Landed the Job	In this chapter, you will discover valuable secrets for becoming a successful pharmacy technician. You will learn about managing important work relationships, how to stay on top of changes in pharmacology and the health care industry, how to manage your time, and how to maximize your built-in mentor—the pharmacist under whose supervision you work.

Appendix A Professional Associations	This is a list of organizations dedicated to developing, educating, and supporting pharmacy technicians.
Appendix B Additional Resources	This is a list of helpful books, magazines, and websites that you can use as a reference throughout your career.
Appendix C Education Programs	This is a list of helpful websites for finding pharmacy technician education programs.
Appendix D Sample FAFSA	Federal Application for Free Student Aid.

Using this book, you will find out if a career as a pharmacy technician is for you. Once you've done that, you will be on your way to learn how to become a successful pharmacy technician.

PHARMACY TECHNICIAN
CAREER STARTER

CHAPTER one

THE HOTTEST CAREERS FOR PHARMACY TECHNICIANS

THIS CHAPTER will help you to decide whether or not you truly want to become a pharmacy technician. You will get an overview of the world of pharmacy technicians and learn what makes a successful pharmacy technician, what they do, and where they work. You will also get advice from a number of those already working in the field.

AN OCCUPATION IN DEMAND

According to the United States Department of Labor, employment of pharmacy technicians is expected to grow as fast as the average for all occupations through 2008. One reason is that our population is growing older, and elderly people use more prescription drugs than younger people do. Technology is increasingly playing a part in keeping people—elderly or otherwise—alive and well, and those people often require continued care as they battle chronic conditions. In addition, our population as a whole has seen an increase in medication use due to stunning pharmaceutical advances in recent years for a multitude of health-related issues. However you approach it, an increase in the demand for medication leads to an increase in the demand for pharmaceutical workers. When this demand is combined with the cost-consciousness of insurers, pharmacies, and healthcare programs, you end up with great opportunities for pharmacy technicians.

You may wonder why cost-consciousness has an impact on the demand for pharmacy technicians. The answer is simple. When companies try to save costs, they rely on lower-paid employees to take on as many tasks as possible. In this case, the lower-paid employees are pharmacy technicians who become responsible for many tasks that once were performed solely by pharmacists.

For example, a local pharmacy may find that they are dispensing a substantially larger number of prescriptions each year. The staff is finding itself spread too thin and work is beginning to pile up. It is harder and harder to keep up with reorders and the pharmacist is worried that patient counseling may soon start to suffer. So, they consider hiring another pharmacist to pick up some of the slack. Once they look at the numbers, they realize that the efficient pharmacy technicians on staff could actually be more involved in some of the routine pharmacy tasks. If they increase the responsibilities for those pharmacy technicians, hire another one, and give them all a 15% pay increase, they spend a lot less than they would have to on a full-time pharmacist. In addition, they are able to keep up with the increase in prescriptions. Their problem is solved and the pharmacy technicians are likely to be happy with their pay and responsibility increase.

The bottom line is that as the responsibilities of pharmacy technicians increases, so does the demand. As a prospective pharmacy technician, you benefit from this increasing trend in the number of jobs available.

Fast Facts

The average prescription price in 2000 was $45.79, up from $42.42 in 1999. The average brand name prescription price in 2000 was $65.29, and the average generic price was $19.33

Source: National Association of Chain Drug Stores

WHAT IS A PHARMACY TECHNICIAN?

The definition of a pharmacy technician varies from state to states and, often, from pharmacy to pharmacy. The basic definition, however, is a person who works under the direct supervision of a licensed pharmacist and performs many pharmacy-related functions. The pharmacy-related functions are limited to those that do not require the professional judgment of a licensed pharmacist. Licensed pharmacists are legally responsible for the care and safety of the pharmacy's patients; pharmacy technicians are not. A pharmacy technician must always work under the supervision of a licensed pharmacist. Since the pharmacist is ultimately responsible for the care of the patients, he or she must review all medications before they go out.

Working as a pharmacy technician is a great place to start if you are interested in having a career in the pharmaceutical industry. Starting as a pharmacy technician provides the type of background training that is necessary to become a pharmacist or work elsewhere in the pharmaceutical industry.

Sample Job Description #1

Award-winning hospital seeks a pharmacy technician to prepare and distribute oral and parenteral medication within the hospital under the direct supervision of a licensed pharmacist.

High School diploma or equivalent required. College courses including chemistry, physiology, algebra, and basic computer desired. Registration as a pharmacy technician with the State Board of Pharmacy is required. The National Pharmacy Technician Certification Exam must be completed and passed upon hire or within the first six months of employment. Must be able to speak, read, and write English. Prior hospital and/or outpatient pharmacy technician skills preferred.

This position requires knowledge of medical terminology, medication in both generic and trade names, pharmaceutical calculation, and regulations relating to the practice of pharmacy. Basic computer knowledge is required and candidates must be able to type 30cwpm. Must be able to perform sterile procedures using proper aseptic technique, including use of vertical and horizontal air flow hoods. Excellent oral and written skills are required.

WHAT DO PHARMACY TECHNICIANS DO?

Pharmacy technicians perform a variety of duties ranging from the administrative and clerical, to tasks that were once performed solely by registered pharmacists. Specific responsibilities vary based on the pharmacy type and setting, and scope of practice.

Typical Duties

Although the duties vary, there are typical ones that most pharmacy technicians will perform. Here is a list of the most common duties of pharmacy technicians:

- ▶ assist the pharmacist in labeling and filling prescriptions
- ▶ assist patients when picking up prescriptions
- ▶ assist with outpatient and inpatient dispensing
- ▶ verify that customers receive the correct prescription(s)
- ▶ compound oral solutions, ointments, and creams, and large volumes of intravenous (IV) mixtures
- ▶ prepackage bulk medications and prepare medication inventories
- ▶ prepare chemotherapeutic agents and IV mixtures
- ▶ maintain and set schedules
- ▶ purchasing and billing
- ▶ enter prescriptions into the computer
- ▶ answer the pharmacy phones and screen calls for pharmacists
- ▶ work with insurance carriers to obtain payments and refilling authority
- ▶ order medication

JOB SATISFACTION

Pharmacy technicians tend to fall into one of three camps. Of these, two camps typically report high levels of job satisfaction and one reports lower levels. Pharmacy technicians who view their job as a stepping stone to a career as a pharmacist are likely to describe their satisfaction as fairly high.

They are in learning mode and are working in the environment where they will continue to build their careers. Some of these pharmacy technicians also may be attending a program in preparation for becoming a registered pharmacist. Their day-to-day work experience will help them in that pursuit.

The second camp that reports a high level of job satisfaction consists of pharmacy technicians who have chosen the job as a career. These often are certified pharmacy technicians and technicians who have attended training programs. They are acutely aware of the importance of the pharmaceutical and healthcare arenas and they strive for excellence in their careers.

So, who isn't satisfied with their job as a pharmacy technician? Well, it happens to be those who see themselves as clerks and who have no desire to turn their job into a career. Sometimes, people apply for and get jobs that they just aren't meant to have. This can happen with pharmacy technicians. People who simply are looking for a job may not have the dedication that a career as a pharmacy technician requires.

Chances are if you have picked up this book with the intention of pursuing a career as a pharmacy technician, then you will fall into one of the first two camps. You will quickly adapt to your routines, you will enjoy interacting with many different people, you will desire to always be learning about new techniques, technologies, and medications, and you will find that you are soon succeeding in a rewarding career!

Sample Job Description #2

Independent pharmacy seeks a hard-working, dedicated pharmacy technician to work under the supervision of a licensed pharmacist. Technician will be expected to assist patients and customers, prepare medical prescriptions, maintain patient records, use a cash register, answer phones, inventory the stock room (reorder and restock as necessary), and perform other related duties as required. The technician will be expected to work a rotating schedule with day, evening, and weekend hours.

This position requires a High School diploma or GED and registration as a pharmacy technician with the State Board of Pharmacy.

SALARY AND BENEFITS

Many factors affect salaries in any industry. They include supply and demand, employer size, and geographic location. Pharmacy technician salaries are also affected by the size and type of pharmacy and by the job responsibilities. So, it can be difficult to pinpoint what a typical pharmacy technician salary is. In general, pharmacy technicians achieve the highest salaries in hospitals, followed by grocery stores, and they typically earn the least working in drug stores. Certification and previous experience will impact the pay even further.

Certified pharmacy technicians usually earn more than their noncertified counterparts. When employers hire a certified technician, they know they are getting someone who is serious about being a pharmacy technician and who has proven his or her knowledge by passing the standardized, national exam.

Technicians who work evenings or weekends are often paid "shift differentials" which increases their earnings. For example, a technician working in a clinic may be paid $9.40 per hour for the hours between 7:00 A.M. and 7:00 P.M. For hours beyond that, she may be paid a shift differential of an additional $0.25 per hour. The amount of this pay and how it is determined depends on the pharmacy and if the pharmacy offers it.

Salary Sampler

The table below represents average yearly salaries for pharmacy technicians with up to three years of experience. The information is based on figures from November 2001 for cities across the United States and the national average.

AREA	LOW	MEDIAN	HIGH
Albany, NY	$19,971	$22,566	$27,179
Austin, TX	$18,392	$20,781	$25,030
Atlanta, GA	$19,143	$21,630	$26,052
Birmingham, AL	$18,450	$20,847	$25,108
Fargo, ND	$17,641	$19,933	$24,007
Los Angeles, CA	$21,512	$24,306	$29,275
Louisville, KY	$19,124	$21,608	$26,025
New Haven, CT	$20,568	$23,240	$27,991
Portland, OR	$19,913	$22,500	$27,100
Richmond, VA	$19,066	$21,543	$25,947
The United States	$19,259	$21,761	$26,209

Source: Salary.com

WHAT MAKES A GOOD PHARMACY TECHNICIAN?

A good pharmacy technician is first and foremost someone who is genuinely interested in pharmacy and healthcare. They are dedicated to their vocation and do their best to keep abreast of changes in the pharmaceutical and healthcare industries.

Aside from having strong positive feelings about their careers, successful pharmacy technicians need to have certain skills and characteristics. They must be organized, pay close attention to the details of their work, and be able to perform precise and often repetitive tasks. Dora Henderson, a CPhT at a hospital-based outpatient infusion clinic, believes that a good work ethic is paramount for successful pharmacy technicians. She says that "critical thinking skills, flexibility, creativity, tons of compassion, a desire to strive for excellence, and to 'never stop learning' are all essential qualities."

Sample Job Description #3

Retail pharmacy has an opening for a pharmacy technician with working knowledge of a retail pharmacy. This position requires knowledge of medical terminology, generic and trade names of commonly prescribed drugs, and pharmaceutical calculations. Knowledge and understanding of pharmaceutical laws and regulations is desired. Applicants should have excellent communication skills, the ability to read and interpret physician orders, typing ability, and basic computer-operation skills. High School diploma or GED is required.

THE IMPORTANCE OF TRAINING

As you begin pursuing your career as a pharmacy technician, you may receive conflicting information about training. This is because there are no cut-and-dried standards for pharmacy technicians. Currently, there are few states that require formal training or certification and there are no federal requirements at all. At the same time, many employers are seeking technicians who have completed formal training and/or are certified.

As you read earlier in this chapter, the pharmaceutical industry is growing along with our aging population and advances in pharmaceutical research. Pharmacists often find themselves with limited time and resources to provide extensive on-the-job training to new technicians. Trained and skilled technicians are therefore more appealing job candidates. The fact that they sought out formal training tells employers that they are dedicated to their career. Those who have earned the right to use CPhT, or certified pharmacy technician, further emphasize to employers their commitment to their vocation.

Formal training can be found at hospitals, proprietary schools, vocation/technical colleges, and community colleges. These programs normally require both classroom and laboratory work. A training program will teach you the fundamentals important to being a successful pharmacy technician. In a typical program you are taught:

▶ medical and pharmaceutical terminology
▶ pharmaceutical calculations
▶ record keeping
▶ pharmaceutical techniques
▶ pharmacy law and ethics
▶ medication names, actions, uses, and doses

Many programs require internships where you will put your knowledge to use in a real pharmacy. Internships are often unpaid but they have many other benefits. You learn first hand what it is like to work as a pharmacy technician. You find out what you know and what you still need to learn. You also gain work experience that you can highlight when you are searching for your first job.

You will learn more about education, training programs, and certification in Chapter 2.

Patient Confidentiality

You will hear a great deal about the importance of patient confidentiality as you begin to investigate your pharmacy technician career. It is critical that you understand early on that patient confidentiality is a serious matter. Every patient and customer must be provided with privacy concerning their medical conditions, therapy, prescribed medications, and other personal information. This means that you cannot discuss **any** of these items outside of the pharmacy. Furthermore, this means that you must do your best to ensure that other customers and non-pharmacy staff do not overhear discussions of medical matters. You also must be careful that the information you enter into the computer is secure.

MODEL CURRICULUM FOR PHARMACY TECHNICIAN TRAINING

In 2001, the American Association of Pharmacy Technicians, the American Pharmaceutical Association, the American Society of Health-System Pharmacists, the National Association of Chain Drug Stores, and the Pharmacy Technician Educators Council collaborated on an update of the *Model Curriculum for Pharmacy Technician Training*. In this publication, they have outlined 35 goals for pharmacy technicians. The goals were divided into two groups: Major Areas of Job Responsibility and Foundation Knowledge and Skills.

The associations developed these goals to help educators create and refine their pharmacy technician training and education programs. These goals can help you as you begin preparing for your career to understand the critical importance of training. Knowing what these associations expect of pharmacy technicians also will help you to identify where you need to focus during your training and any internships in which you may participate.

The goals that the associations identified are as follows:

Major Areas of Job Responsibility
1. Assist the pharmacist in collecting, organizing, and evaluating information for direct patient care, medication use review, and department management.

2. Receive and screen prescription/medication orders for completeness and authenticity.
3. Prepare medications for distribution.
4. Verify the measurements, preparation, and/or packaging of medications produced by other technicians.
5. Distribute medications.
6. Assist the pharmacist in the administration of immunizations.
7. Assist the pharmacist in the identification of patients who desire/require counseling to optimize the use of medications, equipment, and devices.
8. Initiate, verify, assist in the adjudication of, and collect payment and/or initiate billing for pharmacy services and goods.
9. Purchase pharmaceuticals, devices, and supplies according to an established purchasing program.
10. Control the inventory of medications, equipments, and devices according to an established plan.
11. Assist the pharmacist in monitoring the practice site and/or service area for compliance with federal, state, and local laws, regulations, and professional standards.
12. Maintain pharmacy equipment and facilities.
13. Assist the pharmacist in preparing, storing, and distributing investigational medication products.
14. Assist the pharmacist in the monitoring of medication therapy.
15. Participate in the pharmacy department's process for preventing medication misadventures.

Foundation Knowledge and Skills

16. Take personal responsibility for assisting the pharmacist in improving direct patient care.
17. Demonstrate ethical conduct in all job-related activities.
18. Maintain an image appropriate for the profession of pharmacy.
19. Resolve conflicts through negotiation.
20. Understand the principles for managing change.
21. Appreciate the need to adapt direct patient care to meet the needs of diversity.

22. Appreciate the benefits of active involvement in local, state, and national technician and other pharmacy organizations.
23. Appreciate the value of obtaining technician certification.
24. Understand the importance of and resources for staying current with changes in pharmacy practice.
25. Communicate clearly when speaking or writing.
26. Maximize work efficiency through the use of technology.
27. Efficiently solve problems commonly encountered in one's own work.
28. Display a caring attitude toward patients in all aspects of job responsibilities.
29. Maintain confidentiality of patient and proprietary business information.
30. Understand direct patient care delivery systems in multiple practice settings.
31. Efficiently manage one's work whether performed alone or as part of a team.
32. Function effectively as a member of the healthcare team.
33. Balance obligations to one's self, relationships, and work in a way that minimizes stress.
34. Understand the use and side effects of prescription and nonprescription medications used to treat common disease states.
35. Assist the pharmacist in assuring the quality of all pharmaceutical services.

Source: American Society of Health-System Pharmacists. Used by permission.

As you progress in your training and the early stages of your career, you should refer to this list of goals to see where you can make improvements in your knowledge and skills.

WHERE DO PHARMACY TECHNICIANS WORK?

There is no one place that pharmacy technicians work. You may be most familiar with technicians in your local community pharmacy, but these professionals work in many different settings. Some of the places where pharmacy technicians are employed include:

- ▶ hospitals
- ▶ retail pharmacies, independent and national chains
- ▶ pharmacies within grocery stores
- ▶ clinics
- ▶ military
- ▶ home healthcare
- ▶ assisted living communities

It is important for you to understand what your options are, but you do not need to know exactly where you want to work right now. There will be time for you to figure out what environment is best for you once you start looking for a job. If you have basic knowledge of where the jobs are, however, you will be ahead of the game once you actually start looking for your job.

Sample Job Description #4

State University Medical Center and world-renowned teaching hospital is currently seeking pharmacy technicians. Requirements include a high school diploma, inpatient pharmacy experience, and knowledge of aseptic technique. Technical training program and/or national certification preferred. This position will require a 40-hour workweek with rotating 8–12 hour shifts, 4–5 days per week. The State University Medical Center offers a highly competitive compensation package and the opportunity to build a career in a progressive environment.

Hospitals

Hospitals can be fascinating places to work, especially if you thrive in a fast-paced atmosphere where your days are filled with a wide variety of tasks. As a hospital pharmacy technician, you will interact primarily with doctors, nurses, and other hospital staff.

Barry Marshall, CPhT, a pharmacy technician at Orlando Regional Medical Center, describes how varied his job is.

"My typical duties include running refill and delivery reports, delivery of those medications to the med stations throughout the hospital, maintenance of the machines, narcotic control, inventory control and ordering, maintenance of the medication rooms on the patient care units, returning discontinued and unused medications to the central pharmacy and appropriate crediting to the patient, IV preparation, including chemotherapy, for final check by the pharmacist, formulary management of the med station, issuing of codes to new employees and updating users, borrowing and lending medications to affiliate hospitals, answering of telephones, monthly pharmacy inspections of all hospital areas, training of new technicians, filling of prescriptions as the labels are printed by the pharmacists before the final check by the pharmacist, and other auxiliary duties deemed necessary by the pharmacy director."

Retail Pharmacies—Independents and Chains

CVS, Rite-Aid, Walgreens, and Eckerd are all examples of chain pharmacies. One of the benefits to working in one of these establishments is that they often offer standardized training for their pharmacy technicians. Your interaction primarily will be with the pharmacist under whom you work and the patients themselves.

Pharmacies within Grocery Stores

Grocery store pharmacies are similar to other retail pharmacies. Some grocery stores have unions that pharmacy technicians may be able to join. By joining a union, you may be entitled to additional benefits and higher pay. When considering employment in a grocery store pharmacy, you may want to investigate whether or not joining a union is an option and, if so, what the dues and requirements are.

Clinics

Clinics exist to serve myriad populations. There are substance abuse clinics, general medical clinics offering low-cost medical care, rehabilitative treatment clinics, and so on. You may wish to specialize in one area, such as substance abuse, and a clinic could provide you with an excellent environment in which to do so. Or, you may be interested in the clinic atmosphere but want to be exposed to a wide range of patients. A general medical clinic would be a good choice for that. In New York State and Florida, for example, the Health Insurance Plan, or HIP, provides medical services in a clinic setting. Here, patients see their primary care physician or specialist, and if he or she prescribes a medication, the on-site pharmacy dispenses it.

Military

There are many opportunities for pharmacy technicians in the military, and for many people the military offers a rewarding career. The benefits are extensive and the job security is high. But joining the military is a big commitment, and before signing up you should carefully consider whether or not military life is for you. You can visit www.armedforcescareers.com to find out more information. This site has a section devoted to helping you weigh the pros and cons of joining the military.

When you begin investigating the military, you will notice that the various branches refer to pharmacy technicians differently. The U.S. Air Force, for example, calls them pharmacy apprentices. The U.S. Army has pharmacy specialists with different skill levels. In this system, an entry-level pharmacy specialist (comparable to a civilian pharmacy technician) has a clear path of advancement.

If you are interested in becoming a pharmacy technician in the military, start by visiting www.armedforcescareers.com and continue by examining the individual branches websites. These are:

- ▶ Air Force: www.airforce.com
- ▶ U.S. Army: www.goarmy.com
- ▶ Marines: www.marines.com
- ▶ Navy: www.navy.com

Home Healthcare

Remember what you learned about cost-containment earlier in this chapter? Well, it applies here, too. One example is that hospitals contain their costs by moving patients into outpatient facilities, including home healthcare and nursing homes (described below). That is one reason why the United States Department of Labor has predicted substantial growth for the home health-care industry over the next few years. In fact, it is expected that by 2008 there will be 60% more jobs for personal and home care aids than there were in 1998. The patients served by home healthcare often are elderly or terminally ill.

Many home care providers are run by larger networks, organizations, or private companies. Examples of these include Apria Healthcare that has a network of 350 branches, community hospice programs, and visiting nurse services. Most of these homecare providers have websites where you can find more information about the types of services offered and employment opportunities.

Fast Facts

Prescription drugs account for approximately 8% of the total health costs in the United States.* In fact, in 2000 people spent more than $100 billion on drugs in the United States. That's double the amount spent in 1990.**

*Source: National Association of Chain Drug Stores

**Source: The New York Times

Assisted Living Communities

This is a growing area for healthcare in general. In fact, the American Association of Homes and Services for the Aging has approximately 5,600 members serving over 1 million elderly people. Facilities that serve an older population can be religious or secular and range from communities specializing in care of patients with Alzheimer's disease to retirement communities where the residents are largely independent, active, and in search of a care-free lifestyle.

To find out more about assisted living communities and working with an older population, start with local communities and nursing homes. Request a brochure to learn about the services offered and ask if they employ pharmacy technicians. Also, you can learn more by visiting online resources, such as www.retirenet.com or www.welcomefunds.com/assisted-living.

Sample Job Description #5

Private, not-for-profit medical center with a total of 1,112 licensed beds has three openings for the position of pharmacy technician. These positions will assist the pharmacist with dispensing, preparation, and packaging of medication by performing the technical aspects of pharmacy practice within the limits of regulated responsibilities. Certificate of completion from a recognized technician-training program (either academic or hospital based) is required. One year of practical experience as a hospital pharmacy technician (minimum of 2,000 hours) may be substituted for the certificate. Current Technician or Intern registration with the State Board of Pharmacy is required.

DO YOU HAVE WHAT IT TAKES TO BE A PHARMACY TECHNICIAN?

As noted above, most successful pharmacy technicians possess certain skills and characteristics. You may have some of them now, and may be lacking in others. Take this quiz to determine if a career as a pharmacy technician is for you.

	Yes	No
Are you a stickler for details?	____	____
Do you have excellent communication skills?	____	____
Do you enjoy working in a team environment?	____	____
Do you take direction from superiors well?	____	____
Can you type accurately?	____	____
Do you have a basic understanding of medical terminology?	____	____
Do you seek out and read pharmaceutical articles in the newspaper and in magazines?	____	____
Do pharmaceutical advances interest you?	____	____

Are you organized?   _____   _____

Do you enjoy precise work?   _____   _____

Can you perform repetitious work accurately?   _____   _____

Do you take pride in having a strong work ethic?   _____   _____

Can you handle standing on your feet for hours?   _____   _____

Do you enjoy helping others?   _____   _____

Can you move easily from task to task?   _____   _____

Do you pay close attention to your personal hygiene?   _____   _____

Have you done well in math classes?   _____   _____

If you answered "yes" to most of these questions, then a career as a pharmacy technician may just be the career for you! If you answered "no" to several questions, you might want to reconsider why you are interested in pursuing this career.

Sample Job Description #6

We are a national leader in health system medication management providing pharmacy management services and medication management consulting programs. We are looking for a pharmacy technician who, under the supervision of a licensed pharmacist, will assist in the various activities of the pharmacy department. Such duties include: maintaining patient records; setting up, packaging, and labeling medication doses; performing designated tasks regarding processing of equipment and supply orders; and preparation of sterile products.

Qualifications:

- college, high school, or GED
- pharmacy technician work experience (will train if applicant is conscientious and communicates a desire to learn)
- effective oral and written communication skills
- aptitude for working with other healthcare professionals

Candidates who have passed the Pharmacy Technician Certification Exam are preferred.

Now that you know what pharmacy technicians do, where they work, and the importance of formal training, you're ready to start working, right? Not so fast! You have more to learn. Take a look at the next chapter to find out what is involved in pharmacy technician training programs. Then, you will be one step closer to realizing your dream job!

THE INSIDE TRACK

Who: Barry Marshall, CPhT
What: Pharmacy Technician, Level III
Where: Orlando Regional Medical Center
                Orlando, Florida

I am a strong advocate of mandatory national technician certification for all technicians in every state, as well as a proponent of a minimal educational requirement for all technicians. As a certified pharmacy technician, I am more respected by pharmacists, since they realize that they are not just working with a person "off the street" who has no knowledge in the pharmacy area. A pharmacist regards me as a vital, second pair of eyes when he or she calculates, for example, stat doses of antibiotics for newborn babies. I am an asset in the retail setting who can wait on customers, which allows the pharmacist to concentrate on his or her job.

As a certified pharmacy technician, the sky is the limit, especially as mandatory national certification and minimal educational requirements become a reality in every state. Pharmacy customers and patients can only benefit from the increased expertise of CPhTs.

Of course, CPhTs are not looking to replace the knowledge or expertise of the pharmacist in any way. As a matter of fact, it is very important that the pharmacist answer clinical questions, as CPhTs are not trained to do so. Also, it is important for the CPhT to pick up the nonjudgmental tasks that do not need to be performed by the pharmacist, thus freeing them up to do what they were trained to do—improve the health and positive outcome for individuals with prescribed drug therapy.

I have a very strong passion for the pharmacy technician profession, and I am working hard to make all technicians understand that our profession is not "just a job." We have the lives of our patients, literally, in our hands at all times. We are the right hand of the pharmacist. The more competent and educated the pharmacy technician, the better the quality of care we can ultimately provide to our customers, the patients. The pharmacy technician profession can be a great stepping stone to becoming a pharmacist. As a matter of fact, I feel it should be a mandatory experience for all future pharmacists to understand the value of a pharmacy technician by working side-by-side with one as they prepare for their pharmacist careers.

CHAPTER two

ALL ABOUT PHARMACY TECHNICIAN EDUCATION PROGRAMS

TRAINING AND EDUCATION requirements for pharmacy technicians vary by state and by industry. Many employers prefer formal training and certification, and some states are moving toward requiring both. In this chapter you will learn why formal training is a critical aspect in developing a successful career and how to find the right program for you. You will also learn about certification, what it means, how it benefits you, and how to keep your certification once you have achieved it.

EVEN THOUGH you can become a pharmacy technician without formal training, you should view it as a necessary part of your career development. In plain and simple terms, trained technicians make better technicians. You will be more attractive to employers, happier on the job (because you will know and be able to do more), and will eventually earn more as a trained pharmacy technician than you will as a technician with no formal training. Formalized training and eventual certification also will make you feel more committed to your career, affording you that much more satisfaction in your job.

Many employers offer informal on-the-job training but the fundamental skills necessary to do your job as a pharmacy technician are best learned in a training program. The on-the-job training will allow you to further build your knowledge and skills base.

TYPES OF PHARMACY TECHNICIAN TRAINING PROGRAMS

Once you have decided to pursue your education, you will need to determine what your options are and how to find the program that is right for you. Luckily, you have many options. There are four main categories of training:

1. academic programs offered by colleges and universities
2. training programs offered by technical schools
3. proprietary training programs offered by companies (such as CVS)
4. distance learning programs

Each type of training program is discussed further in the next section.

Academic Programs Offered by Colleges and Universities

There are literally thousands of colleges and universities in the United States. Narrowing those down to the one that is right for you can be a daunting task. For now, though, you will need to focus on whether you wish to attend a two-year or four-year program. Most pharmacy technicians choose to pursue a two-year degree rather than a four-year degree, but you should not discount that as an option. There are people who graduate from universities with bachelor's degrees with majors such as chemistry who then go on to make exceptional pharmacy technicians. Whether or not you will choose a four-year program will depend on your interests and your ultimate career goals.

In general, college involves attending regularly scheduled classes and seminars, doing hands-on work in a lab or clinic, completing assignments, and passing exams. For each course you will receive college credit. By completing enough credits, you will earn a degree. To pursue a college degree, a high school diploma or GED is almost always required. Entrance exams, such as the SAT, may also be required. In addition, each school will have application procedures and certain requirements that you will need to fulfill.

The benefit of attending an accredited college or university is that you will graduate with a degree or diploma that will be recognized in any industry—a good safety net if you decide one day that you want to pursue a career other than pharmacy technician. Another benefit is that you will easily be able to further your education in the future, should you choose to do so.

Get Credits in High School

Still in high school? You may be able to receive some college credits by enrolling as a "guest student" at your local community college. If your high school doesn't have a program already in place with a community college, get a copy of the school's course list, and pick out one or two courses that interest you. Then, contact the admissions director. Explain your career plans and interest in sitting in on a course. You will have to pay for it, but in many cases the credit is transferable when you enter college for a degree.

One issue that cannot be underestimated is the significant expense and time commitment involved in attending colleges. Chapter 3 addresses how to pay for your education, once you've decided where you will pursue it. So, you shouldn't let a high price tag dissuade you entirely. As for the time involved in earning a degree, only you can decide how long you are willing to commit.

If time and expense are hurdles, but you know you want to earn a degree, a community college program may be the perfect match for you. Community colleges are especially good if you are interested in a certificate program, will live at home, and work while getting your education. Community colleges are public institutions offering vocational and academic courses both during the day and at night; some community colleges offer two-year degrees (Associate of Arts or Sciences) in addition to certificates. They typically cost less than both two- and four-year public and private institutions.

You can find out the location of community colleges in your area by contacting your state's Department of Higher Education, or use an Internet search engine such as Yahoo.com to find community colleges, which are listed by state. Proprietary schools may also be found on the Internet. Use the search terms "pharmacy technician education" to get started.

Junior colleges are two-year institutions that are usually more expensive than community colleges because they tend to be privately owned. You can earn a two-year degree (AA or AS), which can usually be applied to four-year programs at most colleges and universities. Use the Internet or Peterson's *Two-Year Colleges* to help you with your search.

Colleges and universities that offer four-year programs in which you can earn a bachelor's degree in a variety of fields have entrance requirements that are more stringent than for community colleges; admissions personnel will expect you to have taken certain classes in high school to meet their admission standards. Your high school GPA (grade point average) and standardized test scores (most often the SAT or ACT) will be considered. If your high school grades are weak or it has been some time since you were last in school, you might want to consider taking courses at a community college first. You can always apply to a college or university as a transfer student after your academic track record has improved. Be aware that state or public colleges and universities are often less expensive to attend than private colleges and universities because they receive state funds to offset their operational costs.

Sample Curriculum

COMMUNITY COLLEGE, TWO-YEAR PROGRAM

In a pharmacy technician associate degree program, most of your classes will be required and the majority of those will be in subjects that will directly prepare you for a career as a pharmacy technician. The following sample from Jones County Community College in Mississippi shows a typical curriculum for a two-year program.

Freshman Year—Fall Semester

Pharmacy Technician Fundamentals

Pharmacy Law

Computer Applications in Pharmacy or Introduction to Computer Concepts

Pharmacy Math and Dosage Calculations

Pharmacy Anatomy and Physiology

English Composition I

Freshman Year—Spring Semester

Pharmacology I

Pharmacy Practice

Pharmacy Practice Lab

General Chemistry

Intermediate Algebra

English Composition II

Summer

Practicum I

Pharmaceutical Compounding

Sophomore Year—Fall Semester

Pharmacology II

Oral Communications

Practicum II

Pharmacy Management

Sophomore Year—Spring Semester

Nonprescription Drugs and Devices

Drug Information Research

Practicum III

Pharmacy Transition

Elective

Reprinted with permission of Jones County Community College

Sample Course Description #1: Introduction to Computers

Introduction to computers, hardware and software, including word processing and several different types of pharmacy software for prescription processing, billing, and record storage, drug reference, interaction, and merchandising.

Training Programs Offered by Technical Schools

Technical schools are accredited educational institutions designed for high school graduates looking to earn a degree without having to attend a college or university. They can be perfect programs for people who know that they want to receive specific training for specific careers. They also appeal to those who are looking to obtain the necessary technical training in order to change careers. Technical schools offer the specific courses and training you need to obtain a pharmacy technician degree or certificate.

Most programs take between 8–18 months to complete but there is a wide variance in length between programs. While students are required to attend classes, do hands-on work in labs, complete assignments, and pass exams, most technical schools offer an environment different from that of traditional colleges and universities. The tuition tends to be less expensive but your degree or certificate will show a potential employer that you are knowledgeable and serious about your career, the same way a degree from a two- or four- year school would.

Here are some books that will help you to learn more about vocational and technical schools:

▶ *But What if I Don't Want To Go To College? A Guide to Success Through Alternative Education.* Harlow Giles Unger (New York: Checkmark Books, 1998).

▶ *Peterson's Vocational and Technical Schools West, 4th edition* (Lawrenceville, NJ: Peterson's, 1999).

▶ *You're Certifiable: The Alternative Career Guide to More Than 700 Programs, Trade Schools, and Job Opportunities.* Lee Naftali, and Joel E. Naftali (New York: Fireside, 1999).

There also are websites devoted to vocational and technical school selection. Typing "vocational and/or technical school guide" into a search engine will yield many websites. To get you started, here is a brief list of what is available:

Education World—www.education-world.com
RWM Vocational School Database—www.rmw.org
Vocational Information Center—www.vocationalinformationcenter.
freeservers.com

Sample Curriculum:
Orange Technical Education Centers' Westside Tech (Florida)

Westside Tech's program is innovative and unique in that it requires all students entering the program to pass the Pharmacy Technician Certification Exam (PTCB) Certification Exam in order to receive their Certificate of Completion. The program is based on learning modules and students participate in extensive hands-on training. It offers a day and evening program.

Pharmacy Technician Program—Approximately 1050 hours
The mission of this program is to prepare students for employment as pharmacy technicians. The training includes introduction to medical terminology, medical drugs, pharmaceutical compounding, sterile techniques, maintenance of inventory, IV preparation, delivering medications, prepackaging unit dose packages, patient record systems, control records, preparing purchase orders, receiving and checking supplies purchased, printing labels, typing prescription labels, pricing prescription drug orders and supplies, computer application, employability skills, leadership and human relation skills, health and safety, and CPR.

Pre-Pharmacy Health Careers Core
This program is 90 contact hours. It is required by the State of Florida that all students entering any Health Occupations Program participate in this preliminary program.

Community Pharmacy Practice Skills
Module 205: Practice Human Relations
Module 305: Identify Medical and Legal Considerations
Module 405: Identify Pharmaceutical Abbreviations and Terminology as Related to Community Pharmacy Practice
Module 505: Perform Clerical Duties
Module 605: Demonstrate Knowledge of Basic Pharmaceutical Chemistry and Drug Classification as it Relates to the Human Body's Anatomy
Module 705: Demonstrate Knowledge of Inventory Control

Module 805: Initiate Measurement and Calculating Techniques as it
Relates to Community Practice

Institutional Pharmacy Practice

Module 905: Demonstrate a Basic Knowledge of Pharmaceutical
Chemistry as it Relates to Human Physiology
Module 1005: Prepare and Deliver Medications
Module 1105: Prepackaging Unit Dose Medications
Module 1205: Intravenous Admixtures

Pharmacy Clinical Externship

300 hours total—90 community practice hours and 210 other hours in the
field of choice. (Hospital internship recommended).

Sample Course Description #2: Pharmacy Technician Fundamentals

Introductory course that gives an overview of the pharmacy technician career and
opportunities open to certified pharmacy technicians. Topics discussed include professional literature, the pharmacist-technician relationship, pharmacy ethics, effective communication, brief history of health care and pharmacy, and hospital organization and
department functions. The course is designed to introduce the student to the pharmacy
technician program. One hour lecture. One semester hour credit.

Reprinted with permission of Orange Technical Education Centers' Westside Tech

Proprietary Training Programs

This type of training program typically is offered by an employer to newly
hired employees, or those who have been chosen to enter a particular career
track within the company. Many of the larger national retail pharmacy
chains, hospitals, and other healthcare providers offer training programs for
pharmacy technicians. CVS, for example, has a Pharmacy Support Staff
Training Track to train pharmacy technicians. A proprietary program is perfect for the person who knows where he or she wants to work as a pharmacy technician. They typically involve a commitment on the part of the

student/employee to work for the company while in the training program and for a period of time after the program has been completed.

To investigate your options for this type of program, visit the websites of national retail chains, national healthcare companies, and hospitals where you are interested in working.

Sample Nonproprietary Pharmacy Technician Training Program Description

The Pharmacy Technology program combines classroom instruction with laboratory work and clinical experience to prepare students for employment as technicians. The pharmacy technician works under the supervision of registered pharmacists.

Students learn about pharmacology through an overview of drug classifications, common drug side effects, drug use and abuse, FDA (Food and Drug Administration) testing, and biotransformation of drugs in the human body. The curriculum also includes therapeutic classification of drugs, generic and trade names, transcription abbreviations, and pharmacy math and dosage calculations. The program of study familiarizes the student with methods of drug preparation, packaging and distribution, as well as the functions and services provided by the hospital and retail pharmacy. The program includes practical learning experiences in community settings. Applications for entrance into the program are accepted from January 1 through April 1 each year for acceptance into the class beginning the following August.

Reprinted with permission of Jones County Community College

Distance Learning Program

It's possible to earn a high school diploma or GED, a college degree, a graduate degree, or almost any type of certification by participating in a distance learning program. This means you learn the same material as you would participating in traditional classes but your education is done at home. This allows you to learn at your own pace, through reading, participating in online courses, listening to audiocassettes, and watching videocassettes. If you pass the exams associated with the program, you will earn a degree or certificate just as you would from a traditional educational institution.

Distance learning programs have no residency requirements, allowing students to continue their studies from almost any location. They also typically offer part-time programs and more schedule flexibility. The downside of this flexibility is that if you are not self-motivated you may have trouble sticking with the program.

You can find general information about distance learning programs from these organizations:

American Council on Education
One Dupont Circle
Washington, DC 20036-1193
202-939-9300

Distance Education and Training Council
1601 18th Street, NW
Washington, DC 20009-2529
202-234-5100

National University Continuing Education Association
One Dupont Circle, Suite 615
Washington, DC 20036-1193
202-659-3130

Also, check out the distance learning site at About.com (www. distancelearning.about.com). World Wide Learn (www.worldwidelearn. com/vocational-training.htm) and Degree.net (www.degree.net) are two other Internet resources you can use to learn more. Of course, there are many books available on distance learning, including *Bears' Guide to Earning Degrees by Distance Learning*, 14th edition, by John Bear, Ph.D., and Mariah Bear, M.A. (Berkeley, CA: Ten Speed Press, 2001).

People choose to pursue education through distance learning for many reasons and with recent advances in Internet technology (i.e., streaming audio and video for the Web), distance leaning has been brought to a new level, making it easy to obtain a complete education from any computer with access to the Internet. Distance learning can be an excellent option for someone who already has a job, has limited time available in their daily schedule, or who has financial limitations.

Sample Course Description #3: Pharmaceutical Compounding

This course is a study of the concepts of design, preparation, use, and evaluation of solid and semi-solid dosage forms. Specific topics include powders, tablets, capsules, coated dosage forms, suspensions, emulsions, magmas, gels, lotions, ointments, creams, pastes, suppositories, transdermal systems, sustained release products, and novel drug delivery systems. Exercises in computer application, prescription and physician order interpretation and the introduction of extemporaneous compounding are performed in the laboratory. Two semester hours credit.

Reprinted with permission of Jones County Community College

FINDING THE SCHOOL FOR YOU

Selecting the pharmacy technician training program that will best suit your needs, likes, and goals means making many decisions, including those about the type of school (community college, proprietary school, technical school), overall size of the school, location, and quality of programs. Do you want to go to a local school and live at home, or are you willing to relocate and perhaps live in on-campus housing?

You can explore these options and many others by enlisting the help of an experienced high-school guidance counselor or career counselor. Keep asking questions—of yourself and them—until you have the information you need to make your decision. Talk with people you know who are already working as pharmacy technicians and learn more about their experiences. Ask where they went to school, what advantages they gained from their education, and what they would do differently if they were starting again. You can also ask pharmacies, hospitals, and clinics in your area for recommendations on programs.

Online College Guides

Most of these sites offer similar information, including various search methods, the ability to apply to many schools online, financial aid and scholarship information, and online test taking (PSAT, SAT, etc.). Some offer advice on selecting schools, give virtual campus tours, and help you decide which classes to take in high school. It is well worth it to visit several of them.

www.collegenet.com—On the web since 1995, best for applying to schools online.

www.collegequest.com—Run by Peterson's, a well-known publisher of college guide books (they can also be found at www.petersons.com).

www.collegereview.com—Offers good general information, plus virtual campus tours.

www.embark.com—A good general site.

www.review.com—A service of The Princeton Review. Plenty of "insider information" on schools, custom searches for schools, pointers on improving standardized test scores.

www.theadmissionsoffice.com—Answers your questions about the application process, how to improve your chances of getting accepted, when to take tests.

Evaluating Your Needs

Before making a decision on where to pursue your education, you should consider your needs and the quality of the schools you are interested in. First, make a determination about what you want and need from a pharmacy technician training program in terms of:

▶ location
▶ finances
▶ scheduling

Read through the descriptions of these concerns in the next section, and make notes regarding your position on each of them.

Where to Get Your Training

It makes sense to attend a program located in the geographical area in which you want to work, for a number of reasons. Markets vary even within states, so it's important that you know as much as you can about the area you will be working in. Pharmacy regulations vary from state to state as well. Learning the requirements of your state will be an advantage in your career. Finally, attending school where you will later work allows you to make contacts for future job hunting. Your school may help with job placement locally, and your instructors may be later sources of employment leads. Networking is discussed in greater detail in Chapter 5, but keep in mind that having friends from school when you're out in the job market can be a big help.

What if you're not sure where you are going to end up? You will have to do a little more research to make sure you keep your geographical options open and make the most of the education you do receive. Also, rely on your internships and the faculty of the school you attend. They will most likely be tuned into the pharmacy technician loop and be able to help you find a job once you complete your program. Skilled and knowledgeable pharmacy technicians, with good references from their internships and instructors, are always in demand.

College Guidebooks

Barron's Profiles of American Colleges. **Barron's Educational Series (New York: Barron's, 2001).** This book rates every accredited four-year college and university in the United States. It includes an *Index of Majors*, so you can zero in on those schools offering the program you want.

The Fiske Guide to Colleges 2002. **Edward B. Fiske. Crown (New York: Crown, 2001).** Fiske is the former education editor of the *New York Times*. His guide focuses on the "best and most interesting" 300+ colleges and universities. They are selected on the basis of their academic strength. Also included is a list of "best buys."

The Insider's Guide to the Colleges 2002. **Staff of Yale Daily News (Glendale, CA: Griffin, 2001).**

The most frank of the guides, and the only one researched and written by current college students. There are no statistics, course descriptions, or other bits of "dry" information. What you will find is student-to-student advice on the admissions process, how to choose a school, how to pay for your education, and portraits of the schools that cover many aspects of life on campus, including the condition of the dorms, and the dating scene.

Finances

You are aware of the general differences in costs between each type of school, as touched on briefly above. Now, you will need to think more specifically about what you can afford. While there are many sources of funding for your education (Chapter 3 covers this area in detail), and schools do sometimes offer full or partial scholarships, you will still need to spend some money in order to get quality training. When evaluating the schools you're interested in, be sure to find out all the costs, not just tuition. You will have to purchase books, which can cost hundreds of dollars over the course of the program (and over one thousand dollars if you're considering a bachelor's degree). If you live away from home, you will need to pay for room and board—which can total as much as your tuition at some schools. Will you need childcare while attending classes, or have to drive long distances to get to school? Will you have to buy monthly mass transit passes? Will you have to pay for parking on- or off-campus? How much are student fees? Consider those additional costs when calculating how much you will have to spend.

Don't rule out any schools in which you have an interest at this point. Just be sure to gather as much information as you can about real cost of attendance. Read through Chapter 3 to understand all of your options regarding financing your education. Then, you will be prepared to make an informed decision about which program to attend in terms of what you can afford.

Scheduling

When deciding on a training program, you should think about your schedule and the commitments you may already have made. For instance, do you currently have a job you would like to continue working at while you're in school? You will need to find a program that offers classes at times when you're not working. Will an internship interfere with your employment? It might be a good idea to speak with your employer about your plans and goals. He or she may be willing to offer some flexibility.

If you have young children at home, or some other responsibility that requires your time, consider how you will manage both that responsibility and your education. Some schools offer low-cost childcare to their students. Or perhaps another family member or friend can help while you're attending classes or studying. Be sure to think through all of the potential obstacles to your training and seek out ways to overcome them.

Another option is part-time attendance. If you have young children at home, need to continue working while getting your education, or have another time constraint, part-time attendance can allow you the flexibility your busy schedule demands. But be aware, that while both the financial and time commitments to the program are significantly reduced, it is only for the short term. In the end, you will have spent the same, or more, time and money getting your degree or certificate.

When you've considered what you want in terms the type of program, location, costs, and scheduling, you will be able to make a decision about the type of school to attend. Now, you will need to evaluate those schools that meet your criteria in order to find the one that best suits your needs.

How to Evaluate Training Programs

Since there is no national standard for pharmacy technician education, it can be difficult to compare programs academically. However, there are some national organizations that provide guidelines that may be helpful to you. The *Model Curriculum for Pharmacy Technician Training* excerpted on pages 9–11 of Chapter 1 is a good place to start. When reviewing the curriculum of a school that interests you, keep those goals in mind. You also can visit the websites of the many pharmacy technician associations for their guidelines.

You also should investigate the Pharmacy Technician Certification Board's website (www.ptcb.org) to learn what they require pharmacy technicians to know in order to pass the Pharmacy Technician Certification Exam. You will want to ensure that your program covers all of the important topics so that you will be able to pass the exam and become a certified pharmacy technician.

Keep in mind that schools are businesses; they need students in order to make money. When you think of it in this light, the brochure you read about a school is actually an advertisement. You, as a consumer, need to carefully research, evaluate, and compare schools the same way you would if you were buying a car or major appliance.

Come up with a list of criteria for judging a school or training program's worth to you. For instance, do you want to attend classes full-time or part-time? Are you more comfortable in a rural or urban setting? What kind of student–instructor ratio are you looking for? All of this information is available through a number of sources, including the schools themselves. Make a chart like the one below to help you compare the choices and make your decision.

My Criteria	School A	School B	School C	School D
Urban setting	X	X		
Internship required	X			X
Student-to-instructor ratio less than 10 to 1		X		X
Financial aid offered through the school			X	
8-month program		X	X	

Visiting Schools

After you have found a school (or more than one) that meets your criteria, you should arrange for a visit. Look for cleanliness and organization in the labs. Take note of the students and instructors. Do the students appear engaged and attentive to the instructors?

You also can arrange to sit in on classes for a day if the school allows it. This is called auditing. College students do it all the time—why shouldn't you? Spending some real class time at a school can give you a good idea of what your days would be like, what the students are like, and what the school is really like.

QUESTIONS TO ASK ABOUT TRAINING PROGRAMS

Prospective students need to ask lots of questions in order to ensure they are applying to the right program. Specific questions that you will want to have answered are listed below.

What is the reputation of the institution and the pharmacy technician program?

You want your program to be held in high regard by the pharmacy technician community and the general public. Check with local pharmacy technicians, your guidance counselor, and people you know in the community for more information.

What services are offered to students?

Assistance should be offered in these areas: Orientation, tutoring, academic counseling, financial aid, career information and counseling, and placement assistance. Information on the placement rate and job satisfaction of graduates should be available.

What facilities are available to students?

Programs should have a library, computer laboratories, and properly furnished classrooms. Facilities should accommodate students with disabilities.

What activities are available to students?

Students should have the opportunity to participate in such activities as honor societies and volunteer work. Information about pharmacy technician associations and continuing education should be available.

What is the content and nature of the curriculum?

Programs should offer an experiential learning component such as an internship, practicum, or clinical experience.

What are the graduation requirements?

You should know all of the graduation requirements—number of courses, amount of time spent in the lab, and any special requirements such as an internship.

What are the backgrounds of the program director and faculty?

Your instructors should have the appropriate academic credentials, such as a pharmacy degree or formal pharmacy technician education; program directors may also have advanced degrees in related areas. Many should have experience as pharmacy technicians. Faculty members should have expertise and experience in the subject areas they teach and experience working with or as pharmacy technicians. Make sure they have regular office hours during which you can meet with them.

What are the fees?

You will easily find information on the tuition—it's likely to appear in the school brochure or website—but what about the fees? What are they for? Are fees billed separately from tuition? What's the refund policy? The financial implications of a particular program are important for you to consider up front.

Is the program accredited?

The accreditation process recognizes schools and programs that provide a level of performance, integrity, and quality to its students and the community. It ensures that these schools conform to a minimum set of standards. The accreditation process is voluntary; accreditation is granted on the basis of the school's curriculum, staff ratios, and other criteria established by the accrediting agencies. Accreditation doesn't attempt to rank or grade the schools, only to accredit them.

So what does that mean to you? Basically, it assures you, and your potential employers, that the school you chose to attend provided valuable courses taught by qualified, licensed instructors. In short, it offers you peace of mind.

Most schools are proud of their accredited status and freely share this information in their printed materials, but you can be sure of their status by asking. You can also contact various accrediting associations to obtain a list of the schools they accredit and the standards they use. Some associations you can look into are:

▶ American Society of Health-System Pharmacists (ASHP)
▶ The International University Accrediting Association
▶ The Accrediting Commission of Career Schools and Colleges of Technology
▶ Accrediting Council for Independent Colleges and Schools
▶ New England Schools and Colleges
▶ Distance Education and Training Council
▶ The Accrediting Council for Continuing Education and Training

The ASHP will be of particular interest to you and you can access their ASHP-Accredited Pharmacy Technician Training Program Directory at www.ashp.org/directories/technician. This directory will provide you with basic information on the accredited programs including address, contact person, program description, type of course work, average lecture class size, average lab class size, faculty, costs, and requirements.

What is the program's length?

You have several choices about the amount of time you spend on your training. Decide in advance how long you want to spend on your training and find a program that meets your needs and budget.

What is the student–instructor ratio?

The student–instructor ratio is a statistic that shows the average number of students assigned to one instructor in a classroom or lab. It is important to know the ratio because a lower student–instructor ratio means that, as a student, you will get more small-group, one-on-one, intense training.

What is the classroom–lab ratio?

The lab (also called clinic or practice) experience—applying your knowledge in a hands-on environment—is a must for a pharmacy technician training program. Evaluate how much of your training time will be spent in the classroom versus the lab. Be cautious about any program that does not include significant lab work.

Is the school's lab up-to-date?

Investigate how the labs in your prospective schools are equipped, maintained, and updated. You need to be sure that you will be working with state-of-the-art equipment. If you are learning with equipment and materials that are far out of date you will be way behind the curve when you begin your career. Part of your responsibility as a pharmacy technician will be to use new pharmacy technology and equipment as it evolves, such as robotic machines for dispensing medications and other automation equipment.

What are the school's job-placement statistics?

Most schools and programs have specific placement offices dedicated to helping you find a job after you have completed your training. Placement offices keep records of what types of jobs their students get. Don't just read the statistics; closely examine them.

Understand the difference between a statistic that shows how many students went on to full-time pharmacy technician jobs and one that shows all jobs, internships, part-time, and full-time combined. Find out how many jobs were found through the placement office and how many jobs students found independently. Even if the school or program does not have a job placement service, you should be able to find out what percent of graduating students find full-time pharmacy technician jobs. Ask the admissions office for more information.

MAXIMIZING YOUR SCHOOL EXPERIENCE

Simply signing up for a training program is step 1. It's important that once you begin expanding your knowledge base and skill set that you get the most out of the education available to you. Following are some tips for getting the most out of the training program you participate in.

Set Goals for Yourself

Setting challenging yet achievable goals for yourself while in school is essential in helping you maintain your career focus. By thinking ahead and deciding what kind of environment you want to work in, you can focus your direction. Use the resources your school offers you.

Get Hands-on Experience

Take advantage of every opportunity to get hands-on experience. Use the lab as much as possible. The best way to get hands-on experience, however, is through an internship. Many training programs include internships as part of their curriculum. Although there are basically three types, all internships are designed as learning experiences, giving the intern exposure to an actual working environment. Internships can be one of the following:

▶ Paid—the intern receives a salary for his/her work
▶ College—the intern is a student, and usually receives college credit for his/her work

▶ Summer—the intern is likely to be a student, who may or may not receive college credit

If your school does not provide help in finding internships, or does not offer credit for them, you can find one for yourself. There are a number of ways in which you can uncover an opportunity, either during the summer, during a semester off, or once you have graduated. If your school hires pharmacists to teach some courses, consider enrolling in those courses. You may be able to make a contact or contacts that could lead to an internship. The Internet is also a good source of information. Three sites that offer listings of internships available nationwide are: www.internships.com, www.internjobs.com, and www.vault.com.

The following books are also excellent resources:

America's Top Internships, 2000 Edition. Mark Oldman (New York: Princeton Review, 1999).

Internship Success: Real-World, Step-by-Step Success on Getting the Most Out of Internships. Marianne Ehrlich Green (New York: McGraw Hill/NTC, 1998).

Peterson's 2002 Internships (Lawrenceville, NJ: Peterson's, 2001).

The Internship Bible 2001. Mark Oldman (New York: Princeton Review, 2000).

When you locate specific internship opportunities, some of the questions you will want to ask include:

▶ How many work hours are required to receive credit?
▶ If applicable, how much does the internship pay?
▶ Will you be graded for your work? If so, by an instructor or the person you work under while you are an intern?
▶ Do you have to arrange your own internship or work through your school?
▶ Does the internship program at your school also require you to attend classes, write a paper, or make a presentation to a faculty member in order to receive credit?
▶ What will your responsibilities be on a day-to-day basis?

▶ Who will you be working for?

▶ Will the internship provide real world work experience that's directly related to your chosen field?

▶ Will your participation in the internship provide you with networking opportunities?

Once you land an internship, consider it an audition for ultimately obtaining a full-time job. Always act professionally, ask questions, follow directions, display plenty of enthusiasm, volunteer to take on additional responsibilities, meet deadlines, and work closely with your supervisor. Upon graduating, make sure to highlight your internship work on your resume.

Having an internship on your resume will make you stand out to a recruiter for a number of reasons:

1. You are already familiar with a professional environment and know what is expected of you.
2. You have proven yourself through performance to a potential employer.
3. After evaluating the realities of the job, you are still eager to pursue it.

Take Notes in Class

Very few of us are gifted with a memory that allows us to retain all the information that bombards us throughout each day. And even fewer of us are gifted with a lightning-quick hand that can write down everything that is said in a classroom. So it is essential to your success in a training course that you use an effective note-taking method to help you learn and remember key information. Note taking may not be practical in the lab or clinic setting, but in traditional classroom settings it is critical because your instructors will be imparting important information. Some types of note-taking methods are outlined here.

Traditional Outline

The traditional outline method typically mirrors the way that teachers will lecture. Concepts (broad ideas) are furthest out in the left-hand margin, marked by roman numerals (I, II, III, etc.); the ideas and details that expand the concept are marked first by capital letters (A, B, C, etc.); then Arabic numbers (1, 2, 3, etc.); then lowercase letters (a, b, c, etc.). Increase the indent with each level of detail.

You don't have to get all the lettering and numbering exactly correct. The important part of this method is to understand and accurately record the relationships between the ideas (example: Idea *A* is really a subset of that Idea *I*).

I. How to Make the Most of Your Training Program
   A. Taking Notes
      1. Outline
      2. Shorthand
   B. Studying for Exams

Invent Your Own Shorthand

Writing down every word in a lecture is virtually impossible. You will need to invent ways to abbreviate words. Constantly writing out *medications* and *because* and *training* is just silly (and your wrist will protest). Just *bc* is sufficient for *because*. So many words end with *-ing*, why not just add *-g*? The common ending *-tion* can become *-tn*.

Drop as many vowels as possible without forgetting the meaning of the word. Therefore (and by the way, remember from science class that *therefore* is a triangle of dots?), *training* can easily become *trng*. Use acronyms (just the first letter of each word) for key terms that are repeated over and over. Do you know how many times someone else could write *p.t.* while you're spelling out *Pharmacy Technician?*

You rarely need to write complete sentences. The meat of a sentence is its noun and verb—skip all the extra words (*the*, *it*, etc.). If you haven't tried it before, creating your own shorthand is going to take trial and error, just like any other note-taking method. Experiment with abbreviations while taking down information over the phone. Remember, it's not important that someone else understands your notes, only that *you* understand them.

Review Your Notes

Look over your notes as soon as possible after class—at least within 12 hours. Fill in any missing information that you still remember; cross out what obviously became unimportant by the time the class was done. Mark key points with a highlighter. Make sure each set of notes is clearly titled with date, course title, teacher's name, and overall theme.

Studying for Exams

Contrary to common practice, studying in a group or with your significant other is *not* a good idea. Human nature has a way of reverting to socializing rather than studying. Additionally, if you've perfected your note-taking skills, your friends won't understand the information you've taken in your personal notes anyway. Save your study time for weeknights and save your friends for weekends; that's how the working world is going to be, so you might as well get used to it. You will find that this is the most relaxing set-up of your time in the long run, even if it feels painful in the middle of the week. And it will also prevent the infamous "cram for the exam." Pulling an all-nighter is *not* your red badge of courage in education; it's just plain stupid. Studies show that you will study less effectively and perform worse on the test when you are tired than when you are well-rested and alert.

So, set up a reasonably neat study area and make sure:

- ▶ your lighting is good
- ▶ you have plenty of pens, pencils, Post-it™ notes, and highlighters
- ▶ your telephone isn't going to ring with a tempting offer to go out in lieu of studying
- ▶ you have a comfortable chair and good posture
- ▶ if you prefer listening to music while you study, choose something that will not distract you with song lyrics or bass
- ▶ you have access to a computer that's connected to the Internet. You can use this as a powerful tool for research as well as practicing the hands-on skills you've learned.

Ask your instructor what the format of the exam is going to be: multiple choice, hands-on, or one of the many other methods of testing. You probably won't take many essay exams in your coursework; it's more likely you will encounter multiple-choice and lab (hands-on) tests.

Networking with Other Students

You will be meeting many new people in your training program—take advantage of this great opportunity. There will probably be many students who are in more than one of your classes and they probably have some similar goals and interests. If the program you're in offers social events, take advantage of them as often as you can. Forging friendships with other students can make the transition from student to pharmacy technician easier as well. After graduation, these are the people who may be able to help you get your first job. They may also be your colleagues throughout your career.

Getting to Know Your Instructors

It is important to have peers for moral support and fun, but it's just as important to get to know your instructors. You will discover that instructors are human too. They're not just robotic dispensers of knowledge. So, as soon as you've met one or two times in the classroom, find out your instructors' office hours and location of their offices. Make a point to drop by the office at least twice a month, even if it's just to chat about how things are going for you. Look for notices from student organizations announcing special social times to gather with instructors.

Making the Most of Your Career Placement/Counseling Office

Just think, there are squadrons of people out there who have made it *their job* to run career placement and counseling offices just for you! Take advantage of all their available services. Make the office one of the first places you visit when you set foot on campus, and include it on your list as you're doing rounds to the instructors' offices.

Observe the posters and notices decorating the walls. Ask general questions initially to get a feel for the office; then try to deal with only one person consistently with your specific questions. This will prevent you from becoming just a number—the same strategy you used in getting to know your instructors. If one staff person takes an interest in your situation, they will be able to give you more personalized help and more detailed information.

Not every placement office works in exactly the same way. Get to know the details of how your school's office works. Most offices participate in career fairs and distribute candidate position lists. Career fairs are a great opportunity to learn more about companies in the field and trends in the marketplace, get experience interviewing, and find a job.

CERTIFICATION

Before we get into the details of certification, it is important that you understand that certification—becoming a certified pharmacy technician—is **not** the same as receiving a certificate when you complete a certificate training program; that indicates that you have completed a course of education. Certification in this case means you have passed the Pharmacy Technician Certification Exam (PTCE) and are viewed as having a standard level of competency as a pharmacy technician.

Certification for pharmacy technicians is voluntary, not mandatory. It is required by some states, Texas for instance, and many states are beginning to move toward requiring certification. The Pharmacy Technician Certification Board was created in 1995 by the American Society of Health-Systems Pharmacists, the American Pharmaceutical Association, the Illinois Council of Health-System Pharmacists, and the Michigan Pharmacists Association. The board was developed to be an independent panel to create and administer the national voluntary certification exam. Since the board was created and the exam first given, over 90,000 pharmacy technicians have become certified.

The Pharmacy Technician Certification Exam tests the competency of the candidate to act as a pharmacy technician, with those who pass earning the right to use the title certified pharmacy technician (CPhT). Eligible exam candidates must have a high school diploma or GED. While not required, formal education and/or some experience is extremely helpful to pass the exam.

Certified technicians must be recertified every two years. For recertification, technicians take "CE"—continuing education—courses to stay current in the field. They must complete 20 contact hours of pharmacy related topics within the two-year certification period to be eligible for recertification, with at least one of those hours in the area of pharmacy law. Contact hours can be earned from several different sources including pharmacy associations, pharmacy colleges, and pharmacy technician training programs. Up to ten contact hours can be earned when the technician is employed under the direct supervision and instruction of the pharmacist.

Certification and Salary

A Pharmacy Technician Certification Board survey conducted in 2000 states that "almost 70% of employers give technicians who pass the PTCE a raise." Good incentive to take and pass the exam!

When Should You Take the Exam?

It is best to consider taking the Pharmacy Technician Certification Exam after you complete your training program and have some work experience, from your internship for example. Many training programs recognize the importance of certification so they have made exam preparation part of their curriculum. If that is the case at your program, you will have a distinct advantage when taking the exam; you will be assured that you have the knowledge necessary to pass.

Planning to take the exam soon after you complete your training program is the best situation. The knowledge you have gained from your education will still be fresh and you will be in "study mode" so kicking your studying up a notch for the exam will be relatively easy. You will want to give yourself ample time to prepare for the exam, however, so don't rush into it the day after your program ends. Only you know how long it will take to prepare, based on your habits and study skills. But, consider giving yourself about a month to get ready.

The exam is typically offered four times a year. One of these times should correspond with the end of your program. In 2002, the Pharmacy Technician Certification Exam is offered in January, March, July, and November. Visit their website, www.ptcb.org, to obtain an application and learn about the important deadlines.

Studying For The Exam

Your first step in preparing for your Pharmacy Technician Certification Exam is to visit the Pharmacy Technician Certification Board website at www.ptcb.org. There you will find extensive information on what to expect in your exam and sample questions.

You may wish to purchase other books to help you prepare. There are a number of guides available, a few of which are listed here:

- *APhA's Complete Math Review for the Pharmacy Technician.* American Pharmaceutical Association (Washington, DC: American Pharmaceutical Association, 2001).
- *APhA's Complete Review for the Pharmacy Technician.* American Pharmaceutical Association (Washington, DC: American Pharmaceutical Association, 2001).
- *Delmar's Pharmacy Technician Certification Exam Review.* Patricia K. Anthony (Clifton Park, NY: Delmar, 2000).
- *Drug Information Handbook 2001–2002.* Charles F. Lacy, et al (Hudson, OH: Lexi-Comp, 2001).
- *Pharmacy Math for Technicians.* Don A. Ballington, et al (St. Paul, MN: Paradigm Publishing, 1998).
- *Pharmacy Technician Review and Test Preparation.* Marvin M. Stoogenke (Englewood Cliffs, NJ: Prentice Hall, 1998).
- *Reference Guide for the Pharmacy Technician Exam.* Manan Shroff (Baltimore: Krishna Publishing, 2001).

▶ *The Pharmacy Technician Workbook and Certification Review.* Joseph Medina (Englewood, CO: Morton Publishing and Perspective Press, 1999).

There are many websites that offer certification review including:

▶ www.quicktestprep.com
▶ www.rxtechschool.com
▶ www.coreynahman.com

The exam is well designed, consisting of 125 multiple-choice questions each of which will have one correct or best answer (out of four choices). You are given three hours to complete the exam.

Making a Study Plan

Taking an exam can be a stressful event. When the exam is the national Pharmacy Technician Certification Exam (PTCE), the stress level is even higher. You want to be eligible to use the designation "CPhT" after your name. And, you know that many employers give pharmacy technicians a raise if they pass the PTCE. If you prepare and study well in advance of your exam date, you are sure to reduce your stress. So, you need a study plan that will help you prepare. Follow these directions.

Step 1: Set a Time Frame

Allow yourself plenty of time to study and prepare for the exam.

Step 2: Get the Correct Information

Check filing dates for the test. Double-check your information.

Step 3: Get All Your Materials

Find some review books or other materials you might need to prepare for the test. There are many books available to help you to prepare for the PTCE. If you have access to the Internet, you can find information online.

Step 4: Make a Study Schedule

Plan specific days and times to study and stick to your plan.

Step 5: Stick to Your Plan and Reward Yourself For It

Treat yourself to an afternoon walk, a candy bar, a long phone chat with a friend— anything that will reward you for maintaining a good study schedule. It isn't easy and you should pat yourself on the back when you can stick to your routine for some period of time.

Recertification

As stated above, once you are certified, you must be recertified every two years. To do this, you take continuing education courses—20 contact hours—in pharmacy-related subjects. The Pharmacy Technician Certification Board has outlined the following areas as acceptable subject areas:

▶ medication distribution and inventory control systems
▶ pharmacy administration and management
▶ calculations
▶ programs specific to pharmacy technicians
▶ interpersonal skills
▶ organizational skills
▶ pharmacy law—at least one hour must be in pharmacy law
▶ pharmacology/drug therapy

A maximum of ten hours can be earned at your workplace, but these must be special projects, not your regular work. All of your continuing education must be completed during the two-year recertification period.

You can find continuing education from national pharmacy associations such as The American Pharmaceutical Association, American Society of Health-System Pharmacists, the American Association of Pharmacy Technicians, and many state pharmacy organizations. Your training program may also offer continuing education. Another resource is people with whom you work. If many of them are certified, they will know where the best places for continuing education are.

The Pharmacy Technician Certification Board website is your best resource for all of the details pertaining to certification and recertification. Visit the site before you take the exam, while studying, and many times during your two-year recertification period.

Your pharmacy technician education is the first essential step on the road to your chosen career. Don't view it simply as something to get through, as an ordeal you must overcome before you can begin work and start your real life. School is the time to learn as much about your career and yourself as you possibly can. Along the way, you will make friends and contacts who will be equally valuable to you as you finish school and embark on your career as a pharmacy technician.

THE INSIDE TRACK

Who: Laura Deveau-Diem, CPhT
What: Instructor, Day Program
Where: Westside Tech Pharmacy Technician Training Program
               Winter Park, Florida

I started in Pharmacy in 1978 (I think! It was so long ago!) I was a medical assistant who was not thrilled with the field. I decided it was time for a change so I moved to Boston where I was offered a position as a pharmacy technician. At the time, I did not have a clear idea of what it was, but I liked the concept. I already had a medical background, and I decided that it wouldn't hurt to try this profession. I was certified in May, 1994—I guess it took me a while to learn the trade! But I'm glad I took advantage of the opportunity. Eventually, I made my way down to Florida, and became an instructor at the Westside Tech Pharmacy Training Program in Winter Garden. Now, I love what I do and I especially love sharing my knowledge with future professionals.

My advice for those looking for a good training program includes looking for hands-on training. I have seen programs that say they are hands-on, and in fact just give a quick show-and-tell type of training. I think the student needs to *feel* the work and of course—practice practice, practice!

Prospective students need to ask lots of questions: What will I study? Will I do internships? If so, where? How much time will I spend in the field? Am I required to get a pharmacy job while in class? What kind of teacher-student interaction will there be? I make sure that my students have a one-on-one review with me for every exam. I'm training future colleagues, and I take that seriously.

As far as advice on succeeding in a program, it's simple—the student needs to have a strong desire to work in the field and the drive to commit to the profession. If a student enters the program without those qualities, they will simply not succeed. One of the first things I tell my students is the old cliché: "When you find a job you love, you will never have to work another day in your life." If students understand this, they will make it in the program if they want to. Another important point is that a prospective student needs to understand that retention is the key to pharmacy study. My students may spend a thousand hours with me, but if they do not remember the important facts they learned in the first one hundred hours, they will not be successful in their studies. In order to pass the certification exam, it is essential to retain important facts throughout their education.

When students are seeking employment, my advice is to interview as though it is a lifetime commitment. If you approach the interview as if you may have to spend the rest of your working life with a company, you will come up with interesting and pertinent questions that matter, and relevant and poignant answers to the interviewer's questions that will get you the position.

CHAPTER three

FINANCIAL AID—DISCOVERING THE POSSIBILITIES

IN CHAPTER 2 you learned how to find and succeed in the right training program for you. This chapter explains some of the many different types of financial aid available, gives you information on what financial records you will need to gather to apply for financial aid, and helps you through the process of applying for financial aid. (A sample financial aid form is included in Appendix D.) At the end of the chapter are listed many more resources that can help you find the aid you need.

YOU HAVE decided on a career and you've chosen a training program. Now, you need a plan to finance your training. Perhaps you or your family has been saving for your education, and you've got the money to pay your way. However, if you're like most students, you don't have enough to cover the cost of the training program you'd like to attend. Be assured that it is likely that you can qualify for some sort of financial aid, even if you plan to attend school only part-time.

Because there are many types of financial aid, and the millions of dollars given away or loaned are available through so many sources, the process of finding funding for your education can seem confusing. Read through this chapter carefully, and check out the many resources, including websites and publications, listed in the appendices. You will have a better understanding of where to look for financial aid, what you can qualify for, and how and when to apply.

Also take advantage of the financial aid office at the school you've chosen, or your guidance counselor if you're still in high school. These professionals can offer plenty of information, and can help to guide you through the process. If you're not in school, and haven't chosen a program yet, check the Internet. It's probably the best source for up-to-the-minute information, and almost all of it is free. There are a number of great sites at which you can fill out questionnaires with information about yourself and receive lists of scholarships and other forms of financial aid for which you may qualify. You can also apply for some types of federal and state aid online—you can even complete the Free Application for Federal Student Aid (FAFSA), the basic form that determines federal and state financial aid eligibility, online if you choose.

SOME MYTHS ABOUT FINANCIAL AID

The subject of financial aid is often misunderstood. Here are four of the most common myths:

Myth #1: All the red tape involved in finding sources and applying for financial aid is too confusing for me.
Fact: The whole financial aid process is a set of steps that are ordered and logical. Besides, several sources of help are available. To start, read this chapter carefully to get a helpful overview of the entire process and tips on how to get the most financial aid. Then, use one or more of the resources listed within this chapter and in the appendices for additional help. If you believe you will be able to cope with your training program, you will be able to cope with looking for the money to finance it—especially if you take the process one step at a time in an organized manner.

Myth #2: For most students, financial aid just means getting a loan and going into heavy debt, which isn't worth it, or working while in school, which will lead to burnout and poor grades.
Fact: Both the federal government and individual schools award grants and scholarships, which the student doesn't have to pay back. It is also possible

to get a combination of scholarships and loans. It's worth taking out a loan if it means attending the program you really want to attend, rather than settling for your second choice or not pursuing a career in your chosen field at all. As for working while in school, it's true that it is a challenge to hold down a full-time or even part-time job while in school. However, a small amount of work-study employment (10–12 hours per week) has been shown to actually improve academic performance, because it teaches students important time-management skills.

Myth #3: I can't understand the financial aid process because of all the unfamiliar terms and strange acronyms that are used.
Fact: While you will encounter an amazing number of acronyms and some unfamiliar terms while applying for federal financial aid, you can refer to the acronym list and glossary at the end of this chapter for quick definitions and clear explanations of the commonly used terms and acronyms.

Myth #4: My family makes too much money (or I make too much money), so I shouldn't bother to apply for financial aid.
Fact: The formula used to calculate financial aid eligibility is complex and takes more into account than just your or your family's income. Also, some forms of financial aid—such as a PLUS Loan or an unsubsidized Stafford Loan—are available regardless of calculated financial need. The only way to be certain NOT to get financial aid is to not apply; don't shortchange yourself by not applying, even if you think you won't be eligible.

TYPES OF FINANCIAL AID

There are three categories of financial aid:

1. Grants and scholarships—aid that you don't have to pay back
2. Work-Study—aid that you earn by working
3. Loans—aid that you have to pay back

Each of these types of financial aid will be examined in greater detail, so you will be able to determine which one(s) to apply for and when and how to apply. Note that grants and scholarships are available on four levels: Federal, state, school, and private.

Grants

Grants are normally awarded based on financial need. Even if you believe you won't be eligible based on your own or your family's income, don't skip this section. There are some grants awarded for academic performance and other criteria. The two most common grants, the Pell Grant and the Federal Supplemental Educational Opportunity Grant (FSEOG), are both offered by the federal government.

Federal Pell Grants

Federal Pell Grants are based on financial need and are awarded only to undergraduate students who have not yet earned a bachelor's or professional degree. For many students, Pell Grants provide a foundation of financial aid to which other aid may be added. For the year 2001–2002, the maximum award was $3,750.00. You can receive only one Pell Grant in an award year, and you may not receive Pell Grant funds for more than one school at a time.

How much you get will depend not only on your Expected Family Contribution (EFC) but also on your cost of attendance, whether you're a full-time or part-time student, and whether you attend school for a full academic year or less. You can qualify for a Pell Grant even if you are only enrolled part time in a training program. You should also be aware that some private and school-based sources of financial aid will not consider your eligibility if you haven't first applied for a Pell Grant.

Federal Supplemental Educational Opportunity Grants (FSEOG)

Priority consideration for FSEOG funds is given to students receiving Pell Grants because the FSEOG program is based on exceptional financial need. An FSEOG is similar to a Pell Grant in that it doesn't need to be paid back.

If you are eligible, you can receive between $100 and $4,000 a year in FSEOG funds depending on when you apply, your level of need, and the funding level of the school you're attending. The FSEOG differs from the

Pell Grant in that it is not guaranteed that every needy student will receive one because each school is only allocated a certain amount of FSEOG funds by the federal government to distribute among all eligible students. To have the best chances of getting this grant, apply for financial aid as early as you can after January 1 of the year in which you plan to attend school.

State Grants

State grants are generally specific to the state in which you or your parents reside. If you and your parents live in the state in which you will attend school, you've got only one place to check. However, if you will attend school in another state, or your parents live in another state, be sure to check your eligibility with your state grant agency. Not all states allow their grant money to be used at out-of-state schools. There is a list of state agencies in Appendix A, including telephone numbers and websites, so you can easily find out if there is a grant for which you can apply.

Scholarships

Scholarships are often awarded for academic merit or for special characteristics (for example, ethnic heritage, personal interests, sports, parents' career, college major, geographic location) rather than financial need. As with grants, you do not pay your award money back. Scholarships may be offered from federal, state, school, and private sources.

The best way to find scholarship money is to use one of the free search tools available on the Internet. After entering the appropriate information about yourself, a search takes place which ends with a list of those prizes for which you are eligible. Try www.fastasp.org, which bills itself as the world's largest and oldest private sector scholarship database. A couple of other good sites for conducting searches are www.college-scholarships.com and www.gripvision.com. If you don't have easy access to the Internet, or want to expand your search, your high school guidance counselors or college financial aid officers also have plenty of information about available scholarship money. Also, check out your local library.

To find private sources of aid, spend a few hours in the library looking at scholarship and fellowship books or consider a reasonably priced (under $30) scholarship search service. See the Resources section at the end of this chapter to find contact information for search services and scholarship book titles. Also, contact some or all of the professional associations for the program you're interested in attending; some offer scholarships, while others offer information about where to find scholarships. If you're currently employed, find out if your employer has scholarship funds available. If you're a dependent student, ask your parents and other relatives to check with groups or organizations they belong to as well as their employers to see if they have scholarship programs or contests. Investigate these popular sources of scholarship money:

▶ religious organizations
▶ fraternal organizations
▶ clubs (such as Rotary, Kiwanis, American Legion, Grange, or 4-H)
▶ athletic clubs
▶ veterans' groups (such as Veterans of Foreign Wars)
▶ ethnic group associations
▶ labor unions

If you already know which school you will attend, check with a financial aid administrator (FAA) in the financial aid office to find out if you qualify for any school-based scholarships or other aid. Many schools offer merit-based aid for students with a high school GPA of a certain level or with a certain level of SAT scores in order to attract more students to their school. Check with your program's academic department to see if they maintain a bulletin board or other method of posting available scholarships.

While you are looking for sources of scholarships, continue to enhance your chances of winning one by participating in extracurricular events and volunteer activities. You should also obtain references from people who know you well and are leaders in the community, so you can submit their names and/or letters with your scholarship applications. Make a list of any awards you've received in the past or other honors that you could list on your scholarship application.

Hope Scholarship Credit

Eligible taxpayers may claim a federal income tax credit for tuition and fees up to a maximimum of $1,500.00 per student (the amount is scheduled to be reindexed for inflation after 2002). The credit applies only to the first two years of postsecondary education, and students must be enrolled at least half-time in a program leading to a degree or a certificate. To find out more about the Hope Scholarship Credit, log onto www.sfas.com.

Lifetime Learning Credit

Eligible taxpayers may claim a federal income tax credit for tuition and fees up to a maximimum of $1,000 per student through the year 2002. After the year 2002, eligible taxpayers may claim a credit for tuition and fees up to a maximum of $2,000 per student (unlike the Hope Scholarship Credit, this amount will not be reindexed for inflation after 2002). The Lifetime Learning Credit is not limited to the first two years of postsecondary education; students in any year can be eligible, and there is no minimum enrollment requirement. For more information about the Lifetime Learning Credit, log onto www.sfas.com.

The National Merit Scholarship Corporation

This program offers about 5,000 students scholarship money each year based solely on academic performance in high school. If you are a high school senior with excellent grades and high scores on tests such as the ACT or SAT, ask your guidance counselor for details about this scholarship.

You may also be eligible to receive a scholarship from your state or school. Check with the higher education department of the relevant state or the financial aid office of the school you will attend.

Work-Study Programs

When applying to a college or university, you can indicate that you are interested in a work-study program. Their student employment office will have the most information about how to earn money while getting your education. Work options include the following:

- ▶ on- or off-campus
- ▶ part-time or almost full-time
- ▶ school- or nationally-based

▶ in some cases, in your major (to gain experience) or not (just to pay the bills)

▶ for money to repay student loans or to go directly toward educational expenses

If you're interested in school-based employment, the student employment office can give you details about the types of jobs offered (which can range from giving tours of the campus to prospective students to working in the cafeteria to helping other students in a student service office) and how much they pay.

You should also investigate the Federal Work-Study (FWS) program, which can be applied for on the Free Application for Federal Student Aid (FAFSA). The FWS program provides jobs for undergraduate and graduate students with financial need, allowing them to earn money to help pay education expenses. It encourages community service work and provides hands-on experience related to your course of study, when available. The amount of the FWS award depends on:

▶ when you apply (apply early!)
▶ your level of need
▶ the FWS funds available at your particular school

FWS salaries are the current federal minimum wage or higher, depending on the type of work and skills required. As an undergraduate, you will be paid by the hour (a graduate student may receive a salary), and you will receive the money directly from your school; you cannot be paid by commission or fee. The awards are not transferable from year to year, and not all schools have work-study programs in every area of study.

An advantage of working under the FWS program is that your earnings are exempt from FICA taxes if you are enrolled full-time and are working less than half-time. You will be assigned a job on-campus, in a private non-profit organization, or a public agency that offers a public service. You may provide a community service relating to fire or other emergency service if your school has such a program. Some schools have agreements with private, for-profit companies if the work demands your fire or other emergency skills. The total wages you earn in each year cannot exceed your total FWS award for that year and you cannot work more than 20 hours per week. Your financial aid administrator (FAA) or the direct employer must consider your class schedule and your academic progress before assigning your job.

For more information about National Work Study programs, visit the Corporation for National Service website (www.cns.gov) and/or contact:

National Civilian Community Corps (NCCC)

This AmeriCorps program is an 11-month residential national service program intended for 18–24-year-olds. Participants receive $4,725.00 for college tuition or to help repay education loan debt. Contact: National Civilian Community Corps, 1100 Vermont Avenue NW, Washington, DC 20525, 800-94-ACORPS.

Volunteers in Service to America (VISTA)

VISTA is a part of ACTION, the deferral domestic volunteer agency. This program offers numerous benefits to college graduates with outstanding student loans. Contact: VISTA, Washington, DC 20525, 800-424-8867.

Student Loans

Although scholarships, grants, and work-study programs can help to offset the costs of higher education, they usually don't give you enough money to entirely pay your way. Most students who can't afford to pay for their entire education rely at least in part on student loans. The largest single source of these loans—and for all money for students—is the federal government. However, you can also find loan money from your state, school, and/or private sources. Try these sites for information about federal programs:

www.fedmoney.org

This site explains everything from the application process (you can actually download the applications you will need), eligibility requirements, and the different types of loans available.

www.finaid.org

Here, you can find a calculator for figuring out how much money your education will cost (and how much you will need to borrow), get instructions for filling out the necessary forms, and even information on the various types of military aid (which will be detailed in the next chapter).

www.ed.gov/offices/OSFAP/students

This is the Federal Student Financial Aid Homepage. The FAFSA (Free Application for Federal Student Aid) can be filled out and submitted online. You can find a sample FAFSA in Appendix D, to help familiarize yourself with its format.

www.students.gov

This bills itself as the "student gateway to the U.S. government" and is run as a cooperative effort under the leadership of the Department of Education. You can find information about financial aid, community service, military service, career development, and much more.

You can also get excellent detailed information about different federal sources of education funding by sending away for a copy of the U.S. Department of Education's publication, *The Student Guide*. Write to: Federal Student Aid Information Center, P.O. Box 84, Washington, DC 20044, or call 800-4FED-AID.

Following are some of the most popular federal loan programs.

Federal Perkins Loans

A Perkins Loan has the lowest interest (currently, it's 5%) of any loan available for both undergraduate and graduate students, and is offered to students with exceptional financial need. You repay your school, which lends the money to you with government funds.

Depending on when you apply, your level of need, and the funding level of the school, you can borrow up to $4,000 for each year of undergraduate study. The total amount you can borrow as an undergraduate is $20,000 if you have completed two years of undergraduate study; otherwise, you can borrow a maximum of $8,000.

The school pays you directly by check or credits your tuition account. You have nine months after you graduate (provided you were continuously enrolled at least half-time) to begin repayment, with up to ten years to pay off the entire loan.

PLUS Loans (Parent Loan for Undergraduate Students)

PLUS Loans enable parents with good credit histories to borrow money to pay the education expenses of a child who is a dependent undergraduate student enrolled at least half-time. Your parents must submit the completed forms to your school.

To be eligible, your parents will be required to pass a credit check. If they don't pass, they might still be able to receive a loan if they can show that extenuating circumstances exist or if someone who is able to pass the credit check agrees to co-sign the loan. Your parents must also meet citizenship requirements and not be in default on federal student loans of their own.

The yearly limit on a PLUS Loan is equal to your cost of attendance minus any other financial aid you receive. For instance, if your cost of attendance is $10,000 and you receive $5,000 in other financial aid, your parents could borrow up to, but no more than, $5,000. The interest rate varies, but is not to exceed 9% over the life of the loan. Your parents must begin repayment while you're still in school. There is no grace period.

Federal Stafford Loans

Stafford Loans are low-interest loans that are given to students who attend school at least half-time. The lender is the U.S. Department of Education for schools that participate in the Direct Lending program and a bank or credit union for schools that do not participate in the Direct Lending program. Stafford Loans fall into one of two categories:

Subsidized loans are awarded on the basis of financial need. You will not be charged any interest before you begin repayment or during authorized periods of deferment. The federal government subsidizes the interest during these periods.

Unsubsidized loans are not awarded on the basis of financial need. You will be charged interest from the time the loan is disbursed until it is paid in full. If you allow the interest to accumulate, it will be capitalized—that is, the interest will be added to the principal amount of your loan, and additional interest will be based upon the higher amount. This will increase the amount you have to repay.

There are many borrowing limit categories to these loans, depending on whether you get an unsubsidized or subsidized loan, which year in school you're enrolled, how long your program of study is, and if you're independent or dependent. You can have both kinds of Stafford Loans at the same time, but the total amount of money loaned at any given time cannot exceed $23,000 for a dependent undergraduate student and $46,000 as an independent undergraduate student (of which not more than $23,000 can be in subsidized Stafford Loans). The interest rate varies, but will never exceed 8.25%. An origination fee for a Stafford Loan is approximately 3% or 4% of the loan, and the fee will be deducted from each loan disbursement you receive. There is a six-month grace period after graduation before you must start repaying the loan.

State Loans

Loan money is also available from state governments. In Appendix A you will find a list of the agencies responsible for giving out such loans, with websites and e-mail addresses when available. Remember that you may be able to qualify for a state loan based on your residency, your parents' residency, or the location of the school you're attending.

Alternative Loans

Alternative loans are loans either you, you and a co-borrower, or your parent can take out based on credit; usually the maximum you can borrow is for the cost of education minus all other financial aid received. Interest rates vary but are generally linked to the prime rate. Some of the many lenders who offer these types of loans are listed in the resources section at the end of this chapter. You can also ask your local bank for help or search the Internet for "alternative loans for students."

Questions to Ask Before You Take Out a Loan

In order to get the facts regarding the loan you're about to take out, ask the following questions:

1. What is the interest rate and how often is the interest capitalized? Your college's financial aid administrator (FAA) will be able to tell you this.

2. What fees will be charged? Government loans generally have an origination fee that goes to the federal government to help offset its costs, and a guarantee fee, which goes to a guaranty agency for insuring the loan. Both are deducted from the amount given to you.

3. Will I have to make any payments while still in school? It depends on the type of loan, but often you won't; depending on the type of loan, the government may even pay the interest for you while you're in school.

4. What is the grace period—the period after my schooling ends—during which no payment is required? Is the grace period long enough, realistically, for you to find a job and get on your feet? (A six-month grace period is common.)

5. When will my first payment be due and approximately how much will it be? You can get a good preview of the repayment process from the answer to this question.

6. Who exactly will hold my loan? To whom will I be sending payments? Who should I contact with questions or inform of changes in my situation? Your loan may be sold by the original lender to a secondary market institution, in which case you will be notified as to the contact information for your new lender.

7. Will I have the right to prepay the loan, without penalty, at any time? Some loan programs allow prepayment with no penalty but others do not.

8. Will deferments and forbearances be possible if I am temporarily unable to make payments? You need to find out how to apply for a deferment or forbearance if you need it.

9. Will the loan be canceled ("forgiven") if I become totally and permanently disabled, or if I die? This is always a good option to have on any loan you take out.

APPLYING FOR FINANCIAL AID

Now that you're aware of the types and sources of aid available, you will want to begin applying as soon as possible. You've heard about the Free Application for Federal Student Aid (FAFSA) many times in this chapter already, and should now have an idea of its importance. This is the form used by federal and state governments, as well as schools and private funding sources, to determine your eligibility for grants, scholarships, and loans. The easiest way to get a copy is to log onto www.ed.gov/offices/OSFAP/ students, where you can find help in completing the FAFSA, and then submit the form electronically when you are finished. You can also get a copy by calling 1-800-4-FED-AID, or by stopping by your public library or your school's financial aid office. Be sure to get an original form, because photocopies of federal forms are not accepted.

The second step of the process is to create a financial aid calendar. Using any standard calendar, write in all of the application deadlines for each step of the financial aid process. This way, all vital information will be in one location, so you can see at a glance what needs to be done and when it's due. Start this calendar by writing in the date you requested your FAFSA. Then, mark down when you received it and when you sent in the completed form (or just the date you filled the form out online if you chose to complete the FAFSA electronically). Add important dates and deadlines for any other applications you need to complete for school-based or private aid as you progress though the financial aid process. Using and maintaining a calendar will help the whole financial aid process run more smoothly and give you peace of mind that the important dates are not forgotten.

When to Apply

Apply for financial aid as soon as possible after January 1 of the year in which you want to enroll in school. For example, if you want to begin school in the fall of 2002, then you should apply for financial aid as soon as possible after January 1, 2002. It is easier to complete the FAFSA after you have completed your tax return, so you may want to consider filing your taxes as early as possible as well. Do not sign, date, or send your application before January 1 of the year for which you are seeking aid. If you apply by mail, send your completed application in the envelope that came with the original application. The envelope is already addressed, and using it will make sure your application reaches the correct address.

Many students lose out on thousands of dollars in grants and loans because they file too late. Don't be one of them. Pay close attention to dates and deadlines.

After you mail in your completed FAFSA, your application will be processed in approximately four weeks. (If you file electronically, this time estimate is considerably shorter.) Then, you will receive a Student Aid Report (SAR) in the mail. The SAR will disclose your Expected Family Contribution (EFC), the number used to determine your eligibility for federal student aid. Each school you list on the application may also receive your application information if the school is set up to receive it electronically.

You must reapply for financial aid every year. However, after your first year, you will receive a Student Aid Report (SAR) in the mail before the application deadline. If no corrections need to be made, you can just sign it and send it in.

Getting Your Forms Filed

Follow these three simple steps if you are not completing and submitting the FAFSA online:

1. Get an original Federal Application for Federal Student Aid (FAFSA). Remember to pick up an original copy of this form, as photocopies are not accepted.

2. Fill out the entire FAFSA as completely as possible. Make an appointment with a financial aid counselor if you need help. Read the forms completely, and do not skip any relevant portions or forget to sign the form (or to have your parents sign the form, if required).

3. Return the FAFSA long before the deadline date. Financial aid counselors warn that many students don't file the forms before the deadline and lose out on available aid. Don't be one of those students!

Financial Need

Financial aid from many of the programs discussed in this chapter is awarded on the basis of need (the exceptions include unsubsidized Stafford, PLUS, consolidation loans, and some scholarships and grants). When you apply for federal student aid by completing the FAFSA, the information you report is used in a formula established by the U.S. Congress. The formula determines your Expected Family Contribution (EFC), an amount you and your family are expected to contribute toward your education. If your EFC is below a certain amount, you will be eligible for a Pell Grant, assuming you meet all other eligibility requirements.

There is no maximum EFC that defines eligibility for the other financial aid options. Instead, your EFC is used in an equation to determine your financial needs. Eligibility is a very complicated matter, but it can be simplified to the following equation: your contribution + your parents' contribution = expected family contribution (EFC). Student expense budget/cost of attendance (COA) – EFC = your financial need.

The need analysis service or federal processor looks at the following if you are a dependent student:

▶ Family assets, including savings, stocks and bonds, real estate investments, business/farm ownership, and trusts
▶ Parents' ages and need for retirement income
▶ Number of children and other dependents in the family household
▶ Number of family members in college
▶ Cost of attendance, also called student expense budget, includes tuition and fees, books and supplies, room and board (living with parents, on campus, or off campus), transportation, personal expenses, and special expenses such as childcare

A financial aid administrator calculates your cost of attendance and subtracts the amount you and your family are expected to contribute toward that cost. If there's anything left over, you're considered to have financial need.

Are You Considered Dependent or Independent?

Federal policy uses strict and specific criteria to make this designation, and that criteria applies to all applicants for federal student aid equally. A dependent student is expected to have parental contribution to school expenses; an independent student is not.

You're an independent student if at least one of the following applies to you:

▶ you were born before January 1, 1979 (for the 2002–2003 school year)
▶ you're married (even if you're separated)
▶ you have legal dependents other than a spouse who get more than half of their support from you and will continue to get that support during the award year
▶ you're an orphan or ward of the court (or were a ward of the court until age 18)
▶ you're a graduate or professional student
▶ you're a veteran of the U.S. Armed Forces—formerly engaged in active service in the U.S. Army, Navy, Air Force, Marines, Coast Guard, or as a cadet or midshipman at one of the service academies—released under a condition other than dishonorable. (ROTC students, members of the National Guard, and most reservists are not considered veterans, nor are cadets and midshipmen still enrolled in one of the military service academies.)

If you live with your parents, and if they claimed you as a dependent on their last tax return, then your need will be based on your parents' income. You do not qualify for independent status just because your parents have decided to not claim you as an exemption on their tax return (this used to be the case but is no longer) or do not want to provide financial support for your college education.

Students are classified as *dependent* or *independent* because federal student aid programs are based on the idea that students (and their parents or spouse, if applicable) have the primary responsibility for paying for their postsecondary education. If your family situation is unusually complex and you believe it affects your dependency status, speak to a financial aid counselor at the school you plan to attend as soon as possible. In extremely limited circumstances a financial aid office can make a professional judgment to change a student's dependency status, but this requires a great deal of documentation from the student and is not done on a regular basis. The financial aid office's decision on dependency status is *final* and cannot be appealed to the U.S. Department of Education.

Gathering Financial Records

Your financial need for most grants and loans depends on your financial situation. Now that you've determined if you are considered a dependent or independent student, you will know whose financial records you need to gather for this step of the process. If you are a dependent student, then you must gather not only your own financial records, but also those of your parents because you must report their income and assets as well as your own when you complete the FAFSA. If you are an independent student, then you need to gather only your own financial records (and those of your spouse if you're married). Gather your tax records from the year prior to the one in which you are applying. For example, if you apply for the fall of 2002, you will use your tax records from 2001.

To help you fill out the FAFSA, gather the following documents:

▶ United States Income Tax Returns (IRS Form 1040, 1040A, or 1040EZ) for the year that just ended and W-2 and 1099 forms
▶ records of untaxed income, such as Social Security benefits, AFDC or ADC, child support, welfare, pensions, military subsistence allowances, and veterans' benefits
▶ current bank statements and mortgage information
▶ medical and dental expenses for the past year that weren't covered by health insurance
▶ business and/or farm records
▶ records of investments such as stocks, bonds, and mutual funds, as well as bank Certificates of Deposit (CDs) and recent statements from money market accounts
▶ Social Security number(s)

Even if you do not complete your federal income tax return until March or April, you should not wait to file your FAFSA until your tax returns are filed with the IRS. Instead, use estimated income information and submit the FAFSA, as noted earlier, just as soon as possible after January 1. Be as accurate as possible, knowing that you can correct estimates later.

Maximizing Your Eligibility for Loans and Scholarships

Loans and scholarships are often awarded based on an individual's eligibility. Depending on the type of loan or scholarship you pursue, the eligibility requirements will be different. eStudentLoan.com (www.estudentloan.com/workshop.asp) offers the following tips and strategies for improving your eligibility when applying for loans and/or scholarships:

1. Save money in the parent's name, not the student's name.
2. Pay off consumer debt, such as credit card and auto loan balances.
3. Parents considering going back to school should do so at the same time as their children. Often, the more family members in school simultaneously, the more aid will be available to each.
4. Spend student assets and income first, before other assets and income.
5. If you believe that your family's financial circumstances are unusual, make an appointment with the financial aid administrator at your school to review your case. Sometimes the school will be able to adjust your financial aid package to compensate.
6. Minimize capital gains.
7. Do not withdraw money from your retirement fund to pay for school. If you must use this money, borrow from your retirement fund.
8. Minimize educational debt.
9. Ask grandparents to wait until the grandchild graduates before giving them money to help with their education.
10. Trust funds are generally ineffective at sheltering money from the need analysis process, and can backfire on you.
11. If you have a second home, and you need a home equity loan, take the equity loan on the second home and pay off the mortgage on the primary home.

GENERAL GUIDELINES FOR LOANS

Before you commit yourself to any loans, be sure to keep in mind that they need to be repaid. Estimate realistically how much you will earn when you leave school, remembering that you will have other monthly obligations such as housing, food, and transportation expenses.

Once You're in School

Once you have your loan (or loans) and you're attending classes, don't forget about the responsibility of your loan. Keep a file of information on your loan that includes copies of all your loan documents and related correspondence, along with a record of all your payments. Open and read all your mail about your education loan(s).

Remember also that you are obligated by law to notify both your financial aid administrator (FAA) and the holder or servicer of your loan if there is a change in your:

▶ name
▶ address
▶ enrollment status (dropping to less than half-time means that you will have to begin payment six months later)
▶ anticipated graduation date

After You Leave School

After graduation, you must begin repaying your student loan immediately, or begin after a grace period. For example, if you have a Stafford Loan you will be provided with a six-month grace period before your first payment is due; other types of loans have grace periods as well. If you haven't been out in the working world before, your loan repayment begins your credit history. If you make payments on time, you will build up a good credit rating, and credit will be easier for you to obtain for other things. Get off to a good start, so you don't run the risk of going into default. If you default (or refuse to pay back your loan) any number of the following things could happen to you as a result. You may:

▶ have trouble getting any kind of credit in the future
▶ no longer qualify for federal or state educational financial aid
▶ have holds placed on your college records
▶ have your wages garnished
▶ have future federal income tax refunds taken
▶ have your assets seized

To avoid the negative consequences of going into default in your loan, be sure to do the following:

▶ Open and read all mail you receive about your education loans immediately.
▶ Make scheduled payments on time; since interest is calculated daily, delays can be costly.
▶ Contact your servicer immediately if you can't make payments on time; he or she may be able to get you into a graduated or income-sensitive/income contingent repayment plan or work with you to arrange a deferment or forbearance.

There are a few circumstances under which you won't have to repay your loan. If you become permanently and totally disabled, you probably will not have to (providing the disability did not exist prior to your obtaining the aid) repay your loan. Likewise, if you die, if your school closes permanently in the middle of the term, or if you are erroneously certified for aid by the financial aid office you will probably also not have to repay your loan. However, if you're simply disappointed in your program of study or don't get the job you wanted after graduation, you are not relieved of your obligation.

Loan Repayment

When it comes time to repay your loan, you will make payments to your original lender, to a secondary market institution to which your lender has sold your loan, or to a loan servicing specialist acting as its agent to collect payments. At the beginning of the process, try to choose the lender who offers you the best benefits (for example, a lender who lets you pay electronically, offers lower interest rates to those who consistently pay on time, or who has a toll-free number to call 24 hours a day, 7 days a week). Ask the financial aid administrator at your college to direct you to such lenders.

Be sure to check out your repayment options before borrowing. Lenders are required to offer repayment plans that will make it easier to pay back your loans. Your repayment options may include:

▶ *Standard repayment*: Full principal and interest payments due each month throughout your loan term. You will pay the least amount of interest using the standard repayment plan, but your monthly payments may seem high when you're just out of school.

▶ *Graduated repayment*: Interest-only or partial interest monthly payments due early in repayment. Payment amounts increase thereafter. Some lenders offer interest-only or partial interest repayment options, which provide the lowest initial monthly payments available.

▶ *Income-based repayment*: Monthly payments are based on a percentage of your monthly income.

▶ *Consolidation loan*: Allows the borrower to consolidate several types of federal student loans with various repayment schedules into one loan. This loan is designed to help student or parent borrowers simplify their loan repayments. The interest rate on a consolidation loan may be lower than what you're currently paying on one or more of your loans. The phone number for loan consolidation at the William D. Ford Direct Loan Program is 800-557-7392. Financial aid administrators recommend that you do not consolidate a Perkins Loan with any other loans since the interest on a Perkins Loan is already the lowest available. Loan consolidation is not available from all lenders.

▶ *Prepayment*: Paying more than is required on your loan each month or in a lump sum is allowed for all federally sponsored loans at any time during the life of the loan without penalty. Prepayment will reduce the total cost of your loan.

It's quite possible—in fact likely—that while you're still in school your FFELP (Federal Family Education Loan Program) loan will be sold to a secondary market institution such as Sallie Mae. You will be notified of the sale by letter, and you need not worry if this happens—your loan terms and conditions will remain exactly the same or they may even improve. Indeed, the sale may give you repayment options and benefits that you would not have had otherwise. Your payments after you finish school, and your requests for information should be directed to the new loan holder.

If you receive any interest-bearing student loans, you will have to attend exit counseling after graduation, where the loan lenders or financial aid office personnel will tell you the total amount of debt and work out a payment schedule with you to determine the amount and dates of repayment. Many loans do not become due until at least six to nine months after you graduate, giving you a grace period. For example, you do not have to begin paying on the Perkins Loan until nine months after you graduate. This grace period is to give you time to find a good job and start earning money. However, during this time, you may have to pay the interest on your loan.

If for some reason you remain unemployed when your payments become due, you may receive an unemployment deferment for a certain length of time. For many loans, you will have a maximum repayment period of ten years (excluding periods of deferment and forbearance).

THE MOST FREQUENTLY ASKED QUESTIONS ABOUT FINANCIAL AID

Here are answers to some of the most frequently asked questions about student financial aid:

1. *I probably don't qualify for aid—should I apply for it anyway?*
   Yes. Many students and families mistakenly think they don't qualify for aid and fail to apply. Remember that there are some sources of aid that are not based on need. The FAFSA form is free—there's no good reason for *not* applying.

2. *Do I have to be a U.S. citizen to qualify for financial aid?*

   Students (and parents, for PLUS Loans) must be U.S. citizens or eligible noncitizens to receive federal and state financial aid. Eligible noncitizens are U.S. nationals or U.S. permanent nonresidents (with "green cards"), as well as nonresidents in certain special categories. If you don't know whether you qualify, speak to a financial aid counselor as soon as possible.

3. *Do I have to register with the Selective Service before I can receive financial aid?*

   Male students who are U.S. citizens or eligible noncitizens must register with the Selective Service by the appropriate deadline in order to receive federal financial aid. Call the Selective Service at 847-688-6888 if you have questions about registration.

4. *Do I need to be admitted at a particular university before I can apply for financial aid?*

   No. You can apply for financial aid any time after January 1. However, to get the funds, you must be admitted and enrolled in school.

5. *Do I have to reapply for financial aid every year?*

   Yes, and if your financial circumstances change, you may get either more or less aid. After your first year you will receive a Renewal Application which contains preprinted information from the previous year's FAFSA. Renewal of your aid also depends on your making satisfactory progress toward a degree and achieving a minimum GPA.

6. *Are my parents responsible for my educational loans?*

   No. You and you alone are responsible, unless they endorse or co-sign your loan. Parents are, however, responsible for federal PLUS Loans. If your parents (or grandparents or uncle or distant cousins) want to help pay off your loan, you can have your billing statements sent to their address.

7. *If I take a leave of absence from school, do I have to start repaying my loans?*

   Not immediately, but you will after the grace period. Generally, though, if you use your grace period up during your leave, you will have to begin repayment immediately after graduation, unless you apply for an extension of the grace period before it's used up.

8. *If I get assistance from another source, should I report it to the student finan-cial aid office?*

   Yes—and, unfortunately, your aid amount will possibly be lowered accordingly. But you will get into trouble later on if you don't report it.

9. *Are federal work-study earnings taxable?*

   Yes, you must pay federal and state income tax, although you may be exempt from FICA taxes if you are enrolled full time and work less than 20 hours a week.

10. *My parents are separated or divorced. Which parent is responsible for filling out the FAFSA?*

    If your parents are separated or divorced, the custodial parent is responsible for filling out the FAFSA. The custodial parent is the par-ent with whom you lived the most during the past 12 months. Note that this is not necessarily the same as the parent who has legal cus-tody. The question of which parent must fill out the FAFSA becomes complicated in many situations, so you should take your particular circumstance to the student financial aid office for help.

Financial Aid Checklist

_____ Explore your options as soon as possible once you've decided to begin a training program.

_____ Find out what your school requires and what financial aid they offer.

_____ Complete and mail the FAFSA as soon as possible after January 1.

_____ Complete and mail other applications by the deadlines.

_____ Return all requested documentation promptly to your financial aid office.

_____ Carefully read all letters and notices from the school, the federal student aid processor, the need analysis service, and private scholarship organizations. Note whether financial aid will be sent before or after you are notified about admission, and how exactly you will receive the money.

_____ Gather loan application information and forms from your school or college finan-cial aid office. You must forward the completed loan application to your financial aid office for processing. Don't forget to sign the loan application.

_____ Report any changes in your financial resources or expenses to your financial aid office so they can adjust your award accordingly.

_____ Re-apply each year.

Financial Aid Acronyms Key

COA	Cost of Attendance (also known as COE, Cost of Education)
CWS	College Work-Study
EFC	Expected Family Contribution
EFT	Electronic Funds Transfer
ESAR	Electronic Student Aid Report
ETS	Educational Testing Service
FAA	Financial Aid Administrator
FAF	Financial Aid Form
FAFSA	Free Application for Federal Student Aid
FAO	Financial Aid Office/Financial Aid Officer
FDSLP	Federal Direct Student Loan Program
FFELP	Federal Family Education Loan Program
FSEOG	Federal Supplemental Educational Opportunity Grant
FWS	Federal Work-Study
PC	Parent Contribution
PLUS	Parent Loan for Undergraduate Students
SAP	Satisfactory Academic Progress
SC	Student Contribution
USED	U.S. Department of Education

FINANCIAL AID TERMS—CLEARLY DEFINED

accrued interest—interest that accumulates on the unpaid principal balance of your loan

capitalization of interest—addition of accrued interest to the principal balance of your loan that increases both your total debt and monthly payments

default—failure to repay your education loan

deferment—a period when a borrower, who meets certain criteria, may suspend loan payments

delinquency—failure to make payments when due

disbursement—loan funds issued by the lender

forbearance—temporary adjustment to repayment schedule for cases of financial hardship

grace period—specified period of time after you graduate or leave school during which you need not make payments

holder—the institution that currently owns your loan

in-school grace, and **deferment interest subsidy**—interest the federal government pays for borrowers on some loans while the borrower is in school, during authorized deferments, and during grace periods

interest-only payment—a payment that covers only interest owed on the loan and none of the principal balance

interest—cost you pay to borrow money

lender (originator)—puts up the money when you take out a loan; most lenders are financial institutions, but some state agencies and schools make loans too

origination fee—fee, deducted from the principal, which is paid to the federal government to offset its cost of the subsidy to borrowers under certain loan programs

principal—amount you borrow, which may increase as a result of capitalization of interest, and the amount on which you pay interest

promissory note—contract between you and the lender that includes all the terms and conditions under which you promise to repay your loan

secondary markets—institutions that buy student loans from originating lenders, thus providing lenders with funds to make new loans

servicer—organization that administers and collects your loan; may be either the holder of your loan or an agent acting on behalf of the holder

subsidized Stafford Loans—loans based on financial need; the government pays the interest on a subsidized Stafford Loan for borrowers while they are in school and during specified deferment periods

unsubsidized Stafford Loans—loans available to borrowers, regardless of family income; unsubsidized Stafford Loan borrowers are responsible for the interest during in-school, deferment periods, and repayment

FINANCIAL AID RESOURCES

In addition to the sources listed throughout this chapter, these are additional resources that may be used to obtain more information about financial aid.

Telephone Numbers

Federal Student Aid Information Center (U. S. Department of
Education)

Hotline	800-4-FED-AID
	(800-433-3243)
TDD Number for Hearing-Impaired	800-730-8913
For suspicion of fraud or abuse of federal aid	800-MIS-USED
	(800-647-8733)
Selective Service	847-688-6888
Immigration and Naturalization (INS)	415-705-4205
Internal Revenue Service (IRS)	800-829-1040
Social Security Administration	800-772-1213
National Merit Scholarship Corporation	708-866-5100
Sallie Mae's college AnswerSM Service	800-222-7183
Career College Association	202-336-6828
ACT: American College Testing program	916-361-0656
(about forms submitted to the	
need analysis servicer)	
College Scholarship Service (CSS)	609-771-7725;
TDD	609-883-7051
Need Access/Need Analysis Service	800-282-1550
FAFSA on the Web Processing/Software Problems	800-801-0576

Websites

www.ed.gov/prog_info/SFAStudentGuide
The Student Guide is a free informative brochure about financial aid and is
available on-line at the Department of Education's Web address listed here.

www.ed.gov\prog_info\SFA\FAFSA
This site offers students help in completing the FAFSA.

www.ed.gov/offices/OPE/t4_codes

This site offers a list of Title IV school codes that you may need to complete the FAFSA.

www.ed.gov/offices/OPE/express

This site enables you to fill out and submit the FAFSA on line. You will need to print out, sign, and send in the release and signature pages.

www.career.org

This is the website of the Career College Association (CCA). It offers a limited number of scholarships for attendance at private proprietary schools. You can also contact CCA at 750 First Street, NE, Suite 900, Washington, DC 20002-4242.

www.salliemae.com

This is the website for Sallie Mae that contains information about loan programs.

www.teri.org

This is the website of The Educational Resource Institute (TERI), which offers alternative loans to students and parents.

www.nelliemae.com

This is the website for Nellie Mae; it contains information about alternative loans as well as federal loans for students and parents.

www.key.com

This is Key Bank's website, which has information on alternative loans for parents and students.

www.educaid.com

This is the website for Educaid, which offers both federal and alternative loans to students and parents.

Software Programs

Cash for Class
Tel: 800-205-9581
Fax: 714-673-9039

Redheads Software, Inc.
3334 East Coast Highway #216
Corona del Mar, CA 92625
E-mail: cashclass@aol.com

C-LECT Financial Aid Module
Chronicle Guidance Publications
P. O. Box 1190
Moravia, NY 13118-1190
Tel: 800-622-7284 or 315-497-0330
Fax: 315-497-3359

Peterson's Award Search
Peterson's
P.O. Box 2123
Princeton, NJ 08543-2123
Tel: 800-338-3282 or 609-243-9111
E-mail: custsvc@petersons.com

Pinnacle Peak Solutions (Scholarships 101)
Pinnacle Peak Solutions
7735 East Windrose Drive
Scottsdale, AZ 85260
Tel: 800-762-7101 or 602-951-9377
Fax: 602-948-7603

TP Software—Student Financial Aid Search Software
P.O. Box 532
Bonita, CA 91908-0532
Tel: 800-791-7791 or 619-496-8673
E-mail: mail@tpsoftware.com

Books and Pamphlets

Cassidy, David J. *The Scholarship Book 2002: The Complete Guide to Private-Sector Scholarships, Fellowships, Grants, and Loans for the Undergraduate.* (Englewood Cliffs, NJ: Prentice Hall, 2001).

Chany, Kalman A. and Geoff Martz. *Student Advantage Guide to Paying for College 1997 Edition.* (New York: Random House, The Princeton Review, 1997.)

College Costs & Financial Aid Handbook, 18th ed. (New York: The College Entrance Examination Board, 1998).

Cook, Melissa L. *College Student's Handbook to Financial Assistance and Planning* (City?: Moonbeam Publications, Inc., 1991).

Davis, Kristen. *Financing College: How to Use Savings, Financial Aid, Scholarships, and Loans to Afford the School of Your Choice* (Washington, DC: Random House, 1996).

Hern, Davis and Joyce Lain Kennedy. *College Financial Aid for Dummies* (Foster City, CA: IDG Books Worldwide, 1999).

How Can I Receive Financial Aid for College?

Published from the Parent Brochures ACCESS ERIC website. Order a printed copy by calling 800-LET-ERIC or write to ACCESS ERIC, Research Blvd-MS 5F, Rockville, MD 20850-3172.

Looking for Student Aid

Published by the U.S. Department of Education, this is an overview of sources of information about financial aid. To get a printed copy, call 1-800-4-FED-AID.

Peterson's Scholarships, Grants and Prizes 2002 (Princeton, NJ: Peterson's, 2001).

Ragins, Marianne. *Winning Scholarships for College: An Insider's Guide* (New York: Henry Holt & Company, 1994).

Scholarships, Grants & Prizes: Guide to College Financial Aid from Private Sources. (Princeton, NJ: Peterson's, 1998).

Schwartz, John. *College Scholarships and Financial Aid* (New York: Simon & Schuster, Macmillan, 1995).

Schlacter, Gail and R. David Weber. *Scholarships 2000* (New York: Kaplan, 1999).

The Student Guide

Published by the U.S. Department of Education, this is the handbook about federal aid programs. To get a printed copy, call 1-800-4-FED-AID.

Other Related Financial Aid Books

Annual Register of Grant Support (Chicago, IL: Marquis, annual).

A's and B's of Academic Scholarships (Alexandria, VA: Octameron, annual).

Chronicle Student Aid Annual (Moravia, NY: Chronicle Guidance, annual).

College Blue Book. Scholarships, Fellowships, Grants and Loans (New York: Macmillan, annual).

College Financial Aid Annual (New York: Prentice Hall, annual).

Directory of Financial Aids for Minorities (San Carlos, CA: Reference Service Press, biennial).

Directory of Financial Aids for Women (San Carlos, CA: Reference Service Press, biennial).

Financial Aids for Higher Education (Dubuque, IA: Wm. C. Brown, biennial).

Financial Aid for the Disabled and their Families (San Carlos, CA: Reference Service Press, biennial).

Leider, Robert and Ann. *Don't Miss Out: the Ambitious Student's Guide to Financial Aid* (Alexandria, VA: Octameron, annual).

Paying Less for College (Princeton, NJ: Peterson's, annual).

THE INSIDE TRACK

Who: Donna Estill
What: Pharmacy Technician, CPhT
Where: Northwest Hospital
             Seattle, WA

I am a hospital technician working at Northwest Hospital, in Seattle. I am trained in the IV Room as well as central pharmacy. In Washington State we are fortunate to have strong community college programs and numerous technical college programs. I attended the North Seattle Community College Pharmacy Assistant program and graduated in 1983. It was then a four-quarter program including an externship in hospital and retail settings. In Washington State, this meant I was state-licensed as a "Level A Assistant." That title was gradually changed to "Technician" and that is how Washington State now recognizes us.

I was fortunate to be hired from my extern position as a new graduate from the pharmacy technician program. A couple of years later, when I wanted to move closer to my home, I used the classified ads for my job search because it was in the mid-1980s and Web postings were not the current means of searching for a job. But if I were to go job hunting now, I think that I would print up my resume and actually approach the location where I'd like to work. From experience, I know that hiring can be done without a current position advertised and that good pharmacy technicians are in such short supply that I can virtually select where I want to work.

Originally, I planned to become a pharmacist. Then I realized that the position of technician is a perfect fit for me, and I am quite satisfied with my career choice. I currently work part-time and stay home with my two children part time. I have flexible shifts—working between 8-24 hours each week, on my husband's days off.

Eventually, I earned the additional credits needed to turn my two-year degree into a Bachelor of Arts in Allied Health Sciences. But it wasn't until 2001 that I learned about, took, and passed the National Certification test and finally became certified. For me, the rewards of certification have been more personal than professional. Certification is not a requirement to be employed in Washington State, and there are people who say that it's not necessary. This is true, but I feel that being certified is a testimonial to my dedication to my career choice. I am very glad that such a process is available to help standardize the job classification across the United States.

For people interested in becoming a CPhT, there are multiple study guides, and I encourage working from more than one of them. Job experience is key, as well. If you are not currently employed in a pharmacy, I recommend volunteering in a hospital or retail setting to get as much exposure as you can. There are test questions that may not be covered in a textbook, but by simply being in the pharmacy setting you will know the answer. If one has Internet access, I would also recommend finding the many pharmacy technician websites and forums. This source of education and camaraderie has been very educational and rewarding for me.

More than anything else, the most important qualities needed in a pharmacy technician are attention to detail and a pride in one's work. As with every other career, if you work hard and you are dedicated, you will be fine.

CHAPTER four

HOW TO LAND YOUR FIRST JOB—NETWORKING, AND CONDUCTING YOUR JOB SEARCH

THIS CHAPTER explains how to find the all-important first job after you've completed your training. You will learn how to conduct your job search through networking, research, industry publications, classified ads, online resources, job fairs, and hotlines. Then, in the next chapter, you will learn how to put together a resume and cover letter, and the steps needed to complete successful interviews.

NOW THAT you've completed your pharmacy technician training, you're ready to start looking for a job. Luckily, you can feel confident that you will have many opportunities. According to the U.S. Department of Labor, the job market outlook is great. In their *Occupational Outlook Handbook, 2000-01*, the Bureau of Labor Statistics reports that the pharmacy technician profession will continue to grow as fast as its current average through 2008.

Still, a job search can be a stressful time. After all, you will be spending up to 40 hours or more at your job each week so you should aim to land the type of job you really want, rather than taking the first opportunity that comes along. With many factors to consider during your job search, it can become overwhelming. You can keep from becoming too overwhelmed by preparing before you begin your search and follow-up by being organized during the job search process.

JOB SEARCH PREPARATION

The first step is to make a list of everything that you will need to accomplish during your job search. Here are some essentials to get you started:

▶ *Access to the Internet*—The Internet is one way to research employers so you will want to have access to it. Maybe you have a computer with Internet access at home. If so, you're all set. If not, decide where you will use the Internet: Your local library, your school, or at a relative's home.

▶ *Access to a local newspaper*—The Sunday edition of newspapers have the most extensive Help Wanted sections, so if you are only going to pick up the paper one day each week, pick it up on Sunday.

▶ *Resume paper and envelopes*—You will learn about resume preparation in the next chapter but you should include resume-quality paper on your list of essential job search items.

▶ *A planner*—If you don't already have one, get one now. The type and style is up to you, just be sure that you feel comfortable using it. Some people like a full month on a two-page spread, some people like to see one week per page. Or, you can purchase an electronic device, such as a Palm Pilot™. The planner will be indispensable for helping you keep track of when you sent letters and resumes, made phone calls, and set up interviews. You can also use it to maintain your list of contacts—people you have met while networking who may help you find a job.

▶ *An interview outfit*—It is not essential that you run out and buy a new interview outfit right now. You should start to think about what you will wear if called in for an interview, though. You don't want to find yourself frantically piecing together an outfit after a contact sets up an informational interview for you.

With a complete list of tasks to accomplish, you can set your priorities and estimate how long you think it will take you to accomplish everything on your list. Consider your time estimates to be deadlines and stick to them. Once you have completed everything on your list, you can feel confident that you are prepared for your job search. Now you can relax a little and move on to the next step.

DEVELOPING YOUR PLAN

You're prepared. Now you need a plan. A plan will keep you organized as you progress toward finding your first job. Also it will help you to ensure that your first job is more than just a job. You want your first job to be one that fits into your long-term career plan and will help you to meet your ultimate goals. In order to find that perfect first job, you need to evaluate both your short-term and long-term career goals. To get the job you want, your plan will involve:

1. discovering the kind of job you want
2. conducting a job search
3. developing a resume
4. polishing your cover letter-writing skills
5. learning how to give a great interview
6. understanding which benefits are priorities for you
7. knowing your career options
8. identifying a long-term goal (where you want to be in 5-10-15 years, but knowing that goal can—and probably will—change as you develop in your career)

You can break each of the eight main items on your plan into smaller ones. This will make it easier to accomplish all of the tasks. For example, under #6, you might write:

▶ Find out about typical benefits.
- Ask Mom and Dad about their benefits.
- Look at websites of comparable companies to see what benefits they offer.

▶ Learn about 401k programs.
  ▪ Check out financial websites.
  ▪ Ask Mom about her 401k program.
▶ Think about how much vacation time to expect and what my needs are.
  ▪ Ask friends about their paid vacation benefit.
  ▪ I'm planning my wedding, so I need at least a week for that.

The specifics of your plan will vary depending on your situation. Once you've thought about what is involved in a job search, and written out your plan, you can prioritize it just as you did with your earlier list.

Now, use your planner to create a schedule for yourself. Give yourself deadlines for completing each of the eight main items and all of the sub-items that you have added. Starting at today's date, enter in each job search-related task, one at a time. Leave yourself enough time to accomplish each task, and in your planner, mark down the date by which each task should be completed.

Keep meticulous notes in your planner. Write down everything you do—with whom you make contact, the phone numbers and addresses of your contacts, topics of discussion on the phone or during interviews, the follow-up actions that need to be taken, and even what you wore to each interview. Throughout your job search process, keep your planner with you at all times. Refer to it and update it often to ensure that you remain on track.

Remember to bring your planner with you on job interviews, and don't be afraid to jot down notes during the interview. If the interviewer wants to meet with you again, take out your planner, and make the appointment on the spot. Not only will you be organized, but you will also demonstrate this important quality to a potential employer.

Fast Facts

Pharmacy technicians held approximately 170,000 jobs in 1998, the latest data available.

Source: The United States Department of Labor

Researching Employers

Finding the right job always begins with research. You need to know exactly what jobs you are qualified to fill, what jobs are available, where the jobs can be found, and how to land one of those jobs. You also need to understand that during your job search, you are evaluating the jobs and employers as much as they are evaluating you. You need to research potential employers in order to ensure that the job you find is the right match for you.

Easy ways to research potential employers include asking your instructors and peers what they know about them. Also, if they exist, check out their websites. If possible, pay a visit to see what the job location is like and what type of people work there.

FINDING YOUR JOB

You understand the importance of planning and you've given some thought to what you want out of a career. You've also started to research some of the physical places you could potentially work. Now the question is, just how do you go about finding your first job? Luckily, there are many resources available for the job hunter. And a wise technician-to-be will take advantage of all of them. Just keep in mind that most people apply for many jobs before they are accepted. Don't get discouraged if you send out a dozen resumes and only hear from two pharmacies. That's just part of the process.

Job Search Resources

There are a number of ways to locate employment as a pharmacy technician. Some have been around for years, such as classified ads and job placement firms. Others are more recent additions to the job search arena, and offer great possibilities. They include such Internet resources as industry-specific sites (some of which list employment opportunities) to general career-related websites that furnish everything from tips on writing your resume to links to finding jobs in your area.

Your School

Almost every school has a career placement center, whose director has the job of helping you find employment when you graduate. A good placement office will have directories of employers in the local area, information about job fairs, and copies of any industry publications that list pharmacy technician job openings. A top placement director also maintains contacts with the pharmacy, healthcare, and business communities so that your school's placement office will be one of the first places to hear about a job opening and can give you valuable general information about the market in your area.

Classified Advertising

Conventional job-hunting wisdom says you shouldn't rely too much on classified ads for finding a job. This resource shouldn't be overlooked, however, especially if you're still in school. By reading the classifieds, you can learn valuable information about the market for pharmacy technicians in your area. For instance, you will see at least a partial list of the places that hire pharmacy technicians.

You can get other information from the classifieds, such as typical salaries and benefits in your area. One of the hardest questions to answer on an application or in an interview is "What is your desired salary?" If you've been watching the ads, you will have an idea of the going rate in your area. You can also get information about the temporary and part-time jobs.

Aside from the educational aspect of want ads, reading and responding to them may actually lead to a position. Many employers advertise for pharmacy technicians this way, primarily because it is an inexpensive way to reach a large number of potential applicants. However, that means that, depending on your area, dozens of applicants will send a resume to the employer, and you will be competing with all of them. Don't wait to respond. If the ad appears in the Sunday newspaper, respond to it first thing on Monday morning. Used properly, the classifieds cannot only improve your knowledge of the job market, but can lead to your first position as a pharmacy technician.

If you're looking to move from your current area, check the out-of-town newspapers at your local library, at large bookstores such as Barnes & Noble, or at the newspaper's website. One way to find out-of-town newspaper websites is to visit www.about.com and search for the area where you want to move. If the local newspaper has a website it generally will be listed on the area's About.com website.

When you use the classified ads as a resource, look in the healthcare section of the listings. As with the out-of-town newspapers, you may be able to search your local classified ads online by visiting the website of your daily newspaper.

Sample Job Description #7

The pharmacy technician is the first person most patients see at any pharmacy. This individual is a key member of the Pharmacy Service Support Team, assisting both the pharmacist in dispensing the prescription, and the patient as the first point of contact for any healthcare questions or concerns the patient may have. Becoming a pharmacy technician can be a positive, first step toward a rewarding career in healthcare, and all you need to start is:

- a high school diploma
- a strong background in math and science
- good organizational, communication, and people skills

We provide our pharmacy technicians with the training and educational resources they need to fulfill their responsibilities. You will learn as you work, and we'll prepare you for the Pharmacy Technician Certification Board (PTCB) exam, so you can work as a certified pharmacy technician anywhere in the country. Upon successful completion of the exam, we'll reimburse you the examination fee, and we'll give you a raise!

Career-Related Websites

On the Internet, there are literally thousands of career-related websites. Some of these sites offer "how to" advice about landing a job. Others offer a database of job listings that can be searched by region, industry, job type, salary, position, job title, or almost any other criteria. There are also resume databases allowing applicants to post their resume in hopes of it getting read by a recruiter.

The Internet is an extremely powerful job search tool that can not only help you find exciting job opportunities, but you can also research companies, network with other people in your field, and obtain valuable career-related advice.

Using a Internet Search Engine or portal, such as Google, Yahoo, or Dogpile, for example, you can enter a keyword such as: "resume," "job," "career," "job listings," or "help wanted" to find thousands of websites of interest to you. You can also use a keyword search for "pharmacy technician." The following lists just some of the online resources available to you:

General Online Career Resources

▶ ABA Resume Writing—www.abastaff.com/career/resume/resume.htm
▶ About.com—www.about.com/careers
▶ Accent Resume Writing—www.accent-resume-writing.com/critiques
▶ Advanced Career Systems—www.resumesystems.com/career/Default.htm
▶ America's Job Bank—www.ajb.dni.us
▶ Best Jobs USA—www.bestjobsusa.com
▶ Career Builder—www.careerbuilder.com
▶ Career Center—www.jobweb.org/catapult/guenov/res.html#explore
▶ Career Express—www.careerxpress.com
▶ Career Spectrum—www.careerspectrum.com/dir-resume.htm
▶ CareerMosaic—www.careermosaic.com
▶ CareerNet—www.careers.org
▶ CareerPath—www.careerpath.com
▶ CareerWeb—www.cweb.com
▶ Hot Jobs—www.hotjobs.com
▶ JobBank USA—www.jobbankusa.com
▶ JobSource—www.jobsource.com
▶ Monster Board—www.monster.com
▶ Occupational Outlook Handbook—http://stats.bls.gov/ocohome.htm
▶ Proven Resumes—www.free-resume-tips.com
▶ Resumania—www.resumania.com
▶ USA Jobs—www.usajobs.opm.gov

▶ Salary.com—www.salary.com

▶ Yahoo Careers—www.careers.yahoo.com

Pharmacy Technician Online Career Resources

▶ America's Healthcare Source—www.healthcaresource.com

▶ Healthcare Jobs Online—www.hcjobsonline.com

▶ Hire Health— www.hirehealth.com

▶ Job Science—www.jobscience.com

▶ National Association of Chain Drug Stores—www.nacds.org
    This site links to its members' (Duane Reade, CVS, Eckerd, Walgreen, etc.) career websites.

▶ Nations Job: Medical and Healthcare Jobs Page—www.nationjob. com/medical

▶ Pharmacy Now—www.pharmacynow.org

▶ Pharmacy One Source—www.pharmacyonesrouce.com

▶ Pharmacy Web—www.pharmweb.net

▶ Pharmacy Week—www.pweek.com

▶ RPh On The Go—www.rphonthego.com (jobs for pharm techs)

▶ Rx Career Center—www.rxcareercenter.com

Job Fairs

Attending job or career fairs is another way to find employment. Job fairs bring together a number of employers under one roof, usually at a hotel, convention center, or civic center. These employers send representatives to the fair to inform prospective employees about their company, accept resumes, and, occasionally, to conduct interviews for open positions. Many fairs are held specifically for healthcare employers and prospective employees. They usually hold seminars for attendees covering such topics as resume writing, job hunting strategies, and interviewing skills. To find the next scheduled job fair in your area, contact the information office of the convention center or civic center nearest you and ask if there's a job fair is on their upcoming events calendar. The local newspaper, state unemployment office, or chamber of commerce may have relevant information.

While it's true that you will most likely be competing with many other job seekers at a job fair, your ability to impress an employer is far greater during an in-person meeting than it is if you simply respond to a classified ad by submitting your resume. By attending a job fair, your appearance, level of preparation, what you say and how you say it, as well as your body language can be used to help make an employer interested in hiring you. When attending a job fair, your goal is to get invited to come in later for a formal interview. Since you will have limited time with an employer at a job fair, typically between five and ten minutes, it's very rare that an employer will hire someone on the spot, but this does happen.

Preparation on your part is vital. Determine beforehand which employers will be there and whether or not you have the qualifications to fill the job openings available. Begin your research by visiting the website created to promote the job fair you are interested in attending. The website typically lists detailed information about the employers attending and what types of jobs participating employers are looking to fill. Once you pinpoint the employers you're interested in, research them as if you're preparing for an actual job interview.

Determine exactly how your qualifications and skills meet the needs of employers in which you are interested. Also, develop a list of questions to ask the employer during your in-person meeting at the job fair. Showing a sincere interest in working for an employer and asking questions that demonstrate your interest will help set you apart from the competition in a positive way.

Bring plenty of copies of your resume to the job fair. Begin your visit to the job fair by visiting the companies you are most interested in working for. It's best to visit these employers as early in the day as possible, since as the day goes on, the people working the job fair tend to get tired and may be less responsive, especially if they have already met with several dozen potential applicants. You should be prepared to answer questions about why you want to work for them and how your skills make you qualified to fill one of the positions the employer has available. As you meet with people, collect business cards and follow up your meetings later that day with a short letter, e-mail, or fax, thanking the person you met with for their time. Use this correspondence to reaffirm your interest in working for that employer.

Sample Job Description #8

National retail pharmacy chain is looking for a licensed pharmacy technician or trainee to assist pharmacist in compounding prescriptions, inputting prescriptions, putting away stock orders, cashiering, and other general pharmacy work. Experience is helpful, but willing to train motivated person. Must have some night and weekend availability and be willing to work around school schedule. Company benefits include: Stock options, profit sharing, healthcare, dental care, and vacation benefits.

Salary: Registered Pharmacy Technician $12.00/hour; Trainee $9.95/hour

Industry Newsletters & Magazines

Knowing how to stay on top of changes in pharmacy and healthcare will help make you a more attractive candidate for any job. One of the best ways to track changes and identify trends in the pharmacy community is by reading newspapers and publications geared toward it. These publications will announce breaking news and explain its significance. Being up-to-date on industry news will help convince potential employers that you will be a valuable asset. Reading industry publications will not only keep you current but also may help you find a job. Some publications include job listings as a service to their members.

Several pharmacy and pharmacy technician associations publish regular newsletters and magazines. If you are already a member of them, you probably receive their publications. Associations and organizations of interest to pharmacy technicians are listed in Appendix A.

The Direct Approach

If you really want to work for a place that has no available positions advertised, you should apply to the pharmacy directly. As Donna Estill, a pharmacy technician at a hospital in Seattle, Washington with over 17 years of experience, mentioned in the last chapter, "If I were to go job hunting now, I think that I would print up my resume and actually approach the location that I'd like to work. I know that hiring can be done without a current position advertised and that good pharmacy technicians are in such short supply that I can virtually select where I want to work."

If you choose the direct approach, print out your resume and your list of references and visit the pharmacy. Ask to talk to the pharmacist (try not to pick a time when there will be a large number of patients dropping off or picking up prescriptions). Tell him or her that you are looking for a pharmacy technician job and would like to investigate potential opportunities there. If you are told that they have no openings, ask if you can leave your resume and references in case an opening arises. Ask for the pharmacist's card or write down his or her name (pay attention to the spelling). Then, thank the pharmacist for talking to you.

When you get home, follow-up with a thank you letter re-explaining your situation, expressing your interest in that pharmacy, and providing one or two reasons why you would make an ideal pharmacy technician there. Enclose another copy of your resume.

While you don't want to rely solely on this "pounding-the-pavement" approach, it can't hurt to contact a potential employer directly. You may just end up with a new job.

NETWORKING

Networking just means getting to know people in the pharmacy and health care industries and maintaining contact with them. Networking relationships can provide many benefits:

▶ mentoring
▶ contacts within a prospective employment company
▶ information about emerging technology
▶ cutting-edge training
▶ information about trends in the industry

Through networking, you may discover an opening in the hidden job market—openings for jobs that are never advertised. These jobs can account for up to 70–80% of all job vacancies. This market exists simply because of the large number of employers who are able to fill positions through word of mouth. Employers often feel that when they hire an employee who comes with a personal recommendation, it is like getting a guarantee. Use this to your advantage.

Networking is easier than it sounds. All you have to do is start talking to people about your interests. Tell everyone you know and meet—from your friends and family members to your dentist—that you are training to become a pharmacy technician. Let them know where you eventually want to work, whether it is a hospital, pharmaceutical company, or retail pharmacy. Then, if they know anyone who might be able to help you in your career, they will know to tell you.

A good place to start networking is during your training program. Your instructors can be great resources for referrals. If you have a favorite instructor or an advisor, let him or her know that you are interested in meeting graduates who are working as pharmacy technicians. Or, come right out and ask your instructors if they can introduce you to people who may be in a position to hire you.

In addition, you should consider asking your family and friends to introduce you to people they know who work as pharmacy technicians, pharmacists, or in other positions in health care, especially if they have experience you can learn from. Your Aunt Jennifer may have a best friend who works at a hospital in a nearby city. That person could be an excellent contact but you might not know about her unless your Aunt Jennifer knows that the two of you may have something in common. Don't discount your peers—consider peers who are energetic, personally motivated, and advancing in their field as good contacts too.

A burgeoning area for networking is the Internet. There are discussion groups run by and dedicated to fostering the vocation of pharmacy technician. One discussion group worth investigating is Pharmacy Island (www.groups.yahoo.com/group/PharmacyIsland).

Expanding Your Contact List

Once you begin networking, you should always be looking for ways to expand your list of contacts. Take advantage of every opportunity to meet and get to know people related to your career. If an experienced pharmacy technician speaks to one of your classes, ask him or her a few questions, then ask if it is okay to contact them again in the future. If it is, ask for a business card or a means by which to contact them. Then follow up the next day with a phone call or e-mail, to thank them or ask an additional question.

Also consider requesting informational interviews at pharmacies or hospitals in your area. An informational interview is an excellent opportunity for you to learn more about different practice settings, gain interview experience, impress a contact that may be able to help you in the future, and better understand what people expect from their employees.

Remember that your contacts' willingness to help you will depend on how you ask. Keep your requests for help brief, conversational, and low-key. Above all, be sincere.

Maintaining Your Contacts

It is important to maintain contacts once you have established them. Try to contact people within two weeks of meeting them. You can ask a question, send a note of thanks or a piece of information related to your conversation with them. This follow-up contact cements your meeting in their minds; they will remember you more readily when you contact them again. If you haven't been in contact with someone for a few months, you might send a note or e-mail about a relevant article you read. For example, if you read an article about ATM-style prescription dispensing machines, you might want to photocopy it and send it to any pharmacists or technicians you have met. This shows your contacts that you are truly interested in the industry and it keeps your name fresh in their minds. If they hear of an opening for someone who is responsible and dedicated, they will think of you.

Organizing Your Contact List

You can maintain your contact list in your planner—whether it is a handheld electronic planner or a traditional bound paper planner. Try to maintain the following pieces of information about each person:

- ▶ name
- ▶ address
- ▶ e-mail address
- ▶ phone number(s)
- ▶ fax number
- ▶ company
- ▶ position/specialty (pharmacist, pharmacy technician, supervisor, instructor)
- ▶ first meeting (where, when, what topics did you discuss?)
- ▶ last contact (when, why, and how)

Fast Facts

In 1999, 501 million visits to physician offices resulted in the patient leaving with direction on some sort of medication therapy. That's over 66% of office visits.

Source: National Center for Health Statistics

As you begin your job hunt, keep in mind that you are not just looking for a job; you're looking for a good job, one you will enjoy and that will challenge you. Once you've finished your training, you have much to offer to any employer. Remember: You're not begging for a job; you're trying to find an employer who will be a match for your skills and talents. The next chapter will walk you through the resume and cover letter creation process. You also will learn how to prepare for your interviews and put your best face forward to really wow 'em!

THE INSIDE TRACK

Who: Steve R. Waller

What: Outpatient Pharmacy Technician

Where: Albany Medical Center Hospital

                  Albany, New York

Before my current job, I worked as a technician for nine years at Merck-Medco in Albany, New York—a mail order pharmacy. I started out at Merck doing data entry work, and eventually Merck-Medco trained me to be a pharmacy technician. Before I worked at Merck, I never considered being a technician; but it seemed like an interesting job. I am not a CPhT, but my training at Merck was very thorough, which was necessary to be successful on the job. I also learned a great deal by talking to the pharmacists and keeping my eyes and ears open. No matter how well you are trained, there is no substitute for experience.

Unfortunately, after working nine years at Merck, the company closed. Luckily for me, I worked directly with a large number of pharmacists there, and I talked with a lot them about where they were going to work after we got laid off, and they were a big help. I knew whom to contact, and got many important phone numbers for people who worked for the pharmacies in the area. Through word of mouth and networking, I got my current job—working as an outpatient pharmacy technician at a local hospital. There are many differences between the two jobs. When I worked in mail order, it was like working in a factory; in my current job, I deal with the public quite a bit, and it's important to be helpful and courteous to them. In the mail order business the patient was never seen—so relating to their problems or concerns was very different. But in either business you need to have a good patient understanding because, after all, they are the ones that are directly affected by your job.

A day's typical duties include counting medications, labeling bottles, and stocking the shelves with drug and non-drug items. I also accept prescriptions from patients, enter patient information into the computer, and order supplies for the pharmacy, as well as ask patients if they have any concerns about their medication that the pharmacist can answer for them. Good communication and people skills are a must; you not only need to communicate well with patients, but also with the doctors and your co-workers. A good knowledge of basic types of drugs is also very helpful, because, for example, many times a patient will ask you to fill his blood pressure medication, and you need to know what medication they are talking about, particularly if they are taking more than one.

Being a pharmacy technician can be as satisfying as it is tough. You would think that you are only there to help the pharmacist—which is a true statement—but you have no idea how far that extends. The pharmacist has a very big responsibility to the patient; you need to do everything you can to allow him to focus on that. You need to be sure that the drugs are in stock, in the right place, and that the right information goes to the right patient. There are hundreds of things you need to do to make the pharmacist able to do his or her job well, and you need to be ready to do all of them. You can learn a great deal about drugs and their uses from a pharmacist, and one of my personal satisfactions is being able to see patients improve their quality of life through medication.

I would recommend being a pharmacy technician to anyone who is considering it. The pharmacy technician field is *extremely* diverse and there are so many different opportunities to do different kinds of work—it's up to you to see where you will fit in and excel.

CHAPTER five

RESUMES, COVER LETTERS, AND THE JOB INTERVIEW PROCESS

WRITING YOUR RESUME and cover letters, and promoting yourself in interviews can be stressful, but each can be done well if you prepare in advance. This chapter aims to reduce your job search anxiety by outlining the steps you will need to take to put together a solid resume, craft a professional cover letter, and present a polished and qualified image at your interviews. You will also gain some inside information on what employers look for during interviews.

RESUME AND COVER LETTER BASICS

Once you've identified the job opportunities you plan to pursue, you will need to use a resume and cover letter to apply for those jobs. Combined, these become an extremely important tool for securing interviews and, ultimately, a job. Be sure you take whatever time is necessary to create well thought-out documents that clearly represent who you are and what qualifications you have. Unless you already have met them, potential employers will develop their first impressions of you based on your cover letter and resume.

THE RESUME

A resume is a one-page summary of your qualifications, experience, and interests that you will send to prospective employers. This summary can act as your introduction by mail, or as your calling card if you are applying for a position in person. You don't need to tailor it for each position you apply to, however. That's what a cover letter—a brief note of introduction explaining who you are and why you're interested in a particular position—is for.

The importance of a resume should not be underestimated. It is essential to landing a job as a pharmacy technician, whether you are a new graduate or an experienced, CPhT. The bottom line: A resume proves to potential employers that you are serious about your career as a pharmacy technician and as a professional.

Highlights

Your resume is meant to capture the interest of potential employers, so they will call you for a personal interview. That means your resume should highlight your:

- career objective(s)
- education
- employment history and related experience
- special skills and/or personal qualifications

What Should You Include?

Potential employers all want to know the same basic information about you: Your name/address, education/training, special skills, and work experience. You may also want to include supplemental information such as your career goal/objective, professional organizations to which you belong, activities you participated in, and references.

The dates of your employment and education should be included, as should the titles you held in your various jobs. In the following sections, you will learn the specific information to include on your resume, and how best to organize, format, and word it to make the best possible impression.

Gathering the Information

The following questionnaire will guide you through the information gathering process. By answering the questions, you will have an outline of all the content that should go into each section of your resume. You will also have to think hard about what you want from a job and your career. This will help you get to know yourself better and understand what types of jobs are best for you.

Contact Information

The only personal information that belongs on your resume is your name (on every page, if your resume exceeds one page in length), address, phone number, e-mail, and fax number, if you have one. Under no circumstances should you include personal information such as age, gender, religion, health, marital status, or number of children.

Full name: _____

Permanent Street Address: _____

City, State, Zip: _____

Daytime Telephone Number: _____

Evening Telephone Number: _____

Pager/Cell Phone Number (Optional): _____

Fax Number (Optional): _____

E-Mail Address: _____

Personal Website Address (Optional): _____

School Address (if applicable): _____

_____

Your Phone Number at School (if applicable): _____

Job/Career Objective(s): _____

_____

Write a short description of the job you're seeking. Be sure to include as much information as possible about how you can use your skills to the employer's benefit. Later, you will condense this answer into one short sentence.

_____

_____

_____

_____

What is the job title you're looking to fill? (i.e., pharmacy technician)

_____

Educational Background

Be sure to include any internships in this section. If you are a recent graduate, this may be your only pharmacy experience and perhaps your only work experience. Include the skills you learned which will be applicable to the position for which you're applying.

List the most recent college or university you've attended:_____

City/State:_____

What year did you start?:_____

Graduation month/year:_____

Degree(s), Certificates, and/or Award(s) earned:_____

Your major:_____

Your minor(s):_____

List some of your most impressive accomplishments, extracurricular activities, club affiliations, etc.:_____

_____

List computer courses you've taken that help qualify you for the job you're seeking: _____

_____

_____

Grade point average (GPA):_____

Other college/university, or training program you've attended:_____

_____

City/State:_____

What year did you start?:_____

Graduation month/year:_____

Degree(s), Certificates, and/or Award(s) earned: _____

Your major: _____

Your minor(s): _____

List some of your most impressive accomplishments, extracurricular activities, club affiliations, etc.: _____

_____

List computer courses you've taken that help qualify you for the job you're seeking: _____

_____

_____

Grade point average (GPA): _____

High school attended: _____

City/State: _____

Graduation date: _____

Grade point average (GPA): _____

List the names and phone numbers of one or two current or past professors/teachers (or guidance counselors) you can contact about obtaining a letter of recommendation or list as a reference: _____

_____

_____

_____

Personal Skills and Abilities

Your personal skill set (the combination of skills you possess) is something that differentiates you from everyone else. Skills that are marketable in the workplace aren't always taught in school, however. Your ability to manage people, stay cool under pressure, remain organized, surf the Internet, use software applications, speak in public, communicate well in writing, communicate in multiple languages, or perform research, are all examples of marketable skills.

When reading job descriptions or help wanted ads, pay careful attention to the wording used to describe what the employer is looking for. As you customize your resume for a specific employer, you will want to match up what the employer is looking for with your own qualifications as closely as possible. Try to utilize the wording provided by the employer within the classified ad or job description.

What do you believe is your most marketable skill? Why? _____

_____

_____

_____

List three or four specific examples of how you have used this skill in the past while at work. What was accomplished as a result?

    1. _____

    2. _____

    3. _____

    4. _____

What are keywords or buzzwords that can be used to describe your skill?

_____

_____

_____

What is another of your marketable skills? _____

_____

Provide at least three examples of how you've used this skill in the workplace:

    1. _____

    2. _____

    3. _____

What unusual or unique skill(s) do you possess that help you stand out from other applicants applying for the same types of positions as you?

_____

_____

_____

How have you already proven this skill is useful in the workplace?

_____

What computer skills do you possess? _____

_____

What computer software packages are you proficient in (such as Microsoft Office, Word, Excel, etc.)? _____

_____

Thinking carefully, what skills do you believe you currently lack?

_____

_____

What skills do you have, but need to be polished or enhanced in order to make you a more appealing candidate? _____

_____

What options are available to you to either obtain or brush up on the skills you believe need improvement (for example: evening/weekend classes at a college or university, adult education classes, seminars, books, home study courses, on-the-job-training, etc.)?_____

_____

_____

In what time frame could you realistically obtain this training?

_____

_____

Work/Employment History

Previous work experience is very important. Even unrelated jobs will have taught you something that will make you a better pharmacy technician. Jobs that are related to the one to which you are applying will be considered plusses by potential employers.

Complete the employment-related questions below for all of your previous employers, including part-time or summer jobs held while in school, as well as temporary jobs, internships, and volunteering. You should not reveal your past earning history to a potential employer, but you may want this information available as reference when you begin negotiating your future salary, benefits, and overall compensation package.

Most recent employer:_____

City, State:_____

Year you began work:_____

Year you stopped working (write "Present" if still employed):_____

Job title:_____

Job description:_____

_____

_____

Reason for leaving: _____

_____

_____

What were your three proudest accomplishments while holding this job?

   1. _____

   2. _____

   3. _____

Contact person at the company who can provide a reference: _____

_____

Contact person's phone number: _____

Annual salary earned: _____

Employer: _____

City, State: _____

Year you began work: _____

Year you stopped working (write "Present" if still employed): _____

Job title: _____

Job description: _____

_____

_____

Reason for leaving: _____

_____

_____

What were your three proudest accomplishments while holding this job?

   1. _____

   2. _____

   3. _____

Contact person at the company who can provide a reference: _____

_____

Contact person's phone number: _____

Annual salary earned: _____

Military Service (if applicable)

Branch of service you served in: _____

Years served: _____

Highest rank achieved: _____

Decorations or awards earned: _____

Special skills or training you obtained: _____

Professional Accreditations and Licenses

List any and all of the professional accreditations and/or licenses you have
earned thus far in your career. Be sure to highlight items that directly
relate to the job(s) you will be applying for:

_____

_____

Hobbies and Special Interests

You may have life experience worth pointing out to potential employers. Are
you an EMT? Do you speak fluent Spanish? Many experiences and skills can
add to your attractiveness as a pharmacy technician candidate. If you don't
have a great deal of work experience, this part of your resume is very important. If you can't find a way to include your experiences or special interests
on your resume, mention them in your cover letter.

List any hobbies or special interests you have that are not necessarily work-
related, but can potentially separate you from the competition. Can any
of the skills utilized in your hobby be adapted for the workplace?

_____

_____

What non-professional clubs or organizations do you belong to or actively
participate in? _____

_____

_____

Personal/Professional Ambitions

You may not want to share these on your resume, but answering the questions below will help you to focus your search, and prepare for possible
interviewing topics.

What are your long-term goals?

Personal: _____

_____

_____

Professional: _____

_____

_____

Financial: _____

_____

_____

For your personal, professional, and then financial goals, what are five smaller, short-term goals you can begin working toward achieving right now that will help you ultimately achieve each of your long-term goals?

Short-Term Personal Goals:

1. _____
2. _____
3. _____
4. _____
5. _____

Short-Term Professional Goals:

1. _____
2. _____
3. _____
4. _____
5. _____

Short-Term Financial Goals:

1. _____
2. _____
3. _____
4. _____
5. _____

Will the job(s) you will be applying for help you achieve your long-term goals and objectives? If "yes," how? If "no," why not? _____

_____

_____

_____

Describe your personal, professional, and financial situation right now:

_____

_____

_____

What would you most like to improve about your life overall?_____

_____

_____

What are a few things you can do, starting immediately, to bring about positive changes in your personal, professional, or financial life?_____

_____

_____

_____

Where would you like to be personally, professionally, and financially five and ten years down the road?_____

_____

_____

_____

What needs to be done to achieve these long-term goals or objectives?

_____

_____

_____

_____

What are some of the qualities about your personality that you're most proud of?_____

_____

_____

_____

What are some of the qualities about your personality that you believe need improvement?_____

_____

_____

_____

What do others most like about you?_____

_____

_____

What do you think others least like about you?_____

_____

_____

If you decided to pursue additional education, what would you study and why? How would this help you professionally? _____

_____

_____

_____

If you had more free time, what would you spend it doing? _____

_____

_____

_____

List several accomplishments in your personal and professional life that you're most proud of. Why did you choose these things?

1. _____

2. _____

3. _____

4. _____

5. _____

What were your strongest and favorite subjects in school? Is there a way to incorporate these interests into the job(s) or career path you're pursuing?

_____

_____

_____

_____

What do you believe is your biggest weakness? Why wouldn't an employer hire you? _____

_____

_____

_____

What would be the ideal atmosphere for you to work in? Do you prefer a hospital, clinic, small pharmacy, or retail pharmacy chain?

_____

_____

_____

List five qualities about a particular new job that would make it the ideal employment opportunity for you:

1. _____

2. _____

3. _____

4. _____

5. _____

What did you like most about the last place you worked? _____
_____
_____

What did you like least about the last place you worked? _____
_____
_____

What work-related tasks are you particularly good at? _____
_____
_____

What type of coworkers would you prefer to have? _____
_____
_____

When it comes to work-related benefits and perks, what's most important to
you? _____
_____
_____

When you're recognized for doing a good job at work, how do you like to
be rewarded? _____
_____
_____

If you were to write a help wanted ad describing your ideal dream job, what
would the ad say? _____
_____
_____
_____

Putting It on Paper

Using the information you filled out in the questionnaire, you should be
able to begin writing your resume. For resume wording and formatting, follow the guidelines in this book or purchase one that specifically contains
sample resumes from which you can obtain ideas. Books such as *The*

Pharmacy Professional's Guide to Resumes, CVs, and Interviewing (American Pharmacy Association, 2001) and *Great Resume* by Jason R. Rich (Learning Express, 2000) contain helpful guidelines. And there are plenty of online resources to help you create a winning resume, including the following:

▶ ABA Resume Writing—www.abastaff.com/career/resume/resume.htm
▶ Accent Resume Writing—www.accent-resume-writing.com/critiques
▶ Damn Good Resume—www.damngood.com/jobseekers/tips.html
▶ The Elegant Resume—www.resumeadvice.tripod.com
▶ eResume Writing—www.eresumewriting.com
▶ JobStar—www.jobstar.org/tools/resume
▶ JobWeb—www.jobweb.com/catapult/guenov/restips.html
▶ Learn2 Write a Resume—www.learn2.com/07/0768/0768.asp
▶ Monster.com Resume Center—www.resume.monster.com
▶ Rebecca Smith's eResumes & Resources—www.eresumes.com
▶ Resumania—www.resumania.com
▶ Resume Magic—www.liglobal.com/b_c/career/res.shtml
▶ Resume Tutor—www1.umn.edu/ohr/ecep/resume
▶ Resume Workshop—http://owl.english.purdue.edu/workshops/hypertext/
▶ 10 Minute Resume—www.10minuteresume.com

However you create your resume, never copy it right out of a book. Employers will notice! You can use the sample resumes provided here or in other books as a guide, but the content should be 100% accurate and customized to you.

Start by putting your name, address and telephone number at the top of your resume. If you have an e-mail address, include that, too.

Objective

Under your name and address, you will need to state your job objective, which is your reason for contacting the employer. Under the heading "Objective," describe briefly what you hope to accomplish in your job search, such as "To obtain an entry-level pharmacy technician position at a hospital or medical center."

Education/Training

List the schools you have attended in reverse chronological order, starting with your most recent training, and ending with the least recent. Employers want to be able to see your highest qualifications first. For each educational experience, include dates attended, name and location of school, and degree or certificate earned. If you have not attended college, end with your high school; if you have attended college, it is not necessary to list your high school unless you attended a vocational program.

Work Experience

If you don't have much to list in this section, don't panic. It is not uncommon for people seeking an entry-level pharmacy technician job to have limited work experience. If you do have related work experience, list it in reverse chronological order, just like you listed your education/training. Include company name and location (city, state), the position you held, and the dates of employment. Write a few lines describing the nature of your work.

What if you don't have any related experience yet? List any employment experiences you've had where you've developed the skills and traits needed to become a successful pharmacy technician. Your potential employer is looking to hire someone who is reliable, responsible, pays attention to detail, and understands basic medical terminology.

Special Skills

You may wish to include another section called "Special Skills," "Awards," or "Personal Qualifications." When you do not yet have a lot of experience, this is a section that can help you stand apart from the crowd. Items that you may want to include in this section are:

▶ awards won during your training program
▶ languages (in addition to English) that you speak
▶ special certifications, such as CPR

Resume Creation Tips

These tips and strategies will ensure that your resume makes the most impact possible when a potential employer reads it.

- Always use standard, letter-size paper in ivory, cream, or another neutral color.
- Include your name, address, and phone number on every page.
- Make sure your name is larger than everything else on the page (example: your name in 14-point font, the rest in 12-point).
- Use a font that is easy to read, such as 12-point Times New Roman.
- Do not use more than three fonts in your resume.
- Use bullet points for items in a list—they highlight your main points, making them hard to miss.
- Use key pharmaceutical terms.
- Avoid using excessive graphics, distracting lines, and complex designs.
- Be consistent when using bold, capitalization, underlining, and italics. If one company name is in bold, make sure all are in bold. Check titles, dates, etc.
- Don't list your nationality, race, religion, or gender. Keep your resume as neutral as possible. Your resume is a summary of your skills and abilities.
- Don't put anything personal on your resume such as your birth date, marital status, or height.
- One page is best, but a crowded resume is not. Shorten the margins if you need more space; if it's necessary to create a two-page resume, make sure you balance the information on each page. Don't put just one section on the second page.
- Keep your resume updated. Don't write "4/00 to present" if you ended your job two months ago. Never hand-write changes on your resume.
- Understand and remember everything written on your resume. Be able to back up all statements with specific examples.
- Last, and most important: Edit, edit, edit! Once you've finished your resume, read it over thoroughly checking for consistency, errors, and readability. Then have friends with good proofreading skills, or a teacher or guidance counselor read it. Don't rely heavily on grammar and spell checkers, which can miss errors.

Avoid making these common resume errors:

- **Lying or stretching the truth**—A growing number of employers are verifying all resume information. If you're caught lying, you won't be offered a job, or you could be fired later if it's discovered that you weren't truthful.

- **Including salary references**—Unless an advertisement specifically asks for your salary history or requirements, do not include any past salary information or how much you're looking to earn within your resume and cover letter. If you must include salary requirements, consider stating that you require a salary commensurate with your skills and the nature of the position.

- **Listing the reasons why you switched jobs, or are currently looking for a new job**—Do not include a line in your resume saying, "Unemployed" or "Out of Work" along with the corresponding dates in order to fill a time gap.

- **Having a typo or grammatical error in a resume**—As a pharmacy technician, you will be required to pay extremely close attention to details, especially when reading and filling prescriptions. If you ignore the details on your resume, why should an employer assume you'd take the time needed to do your job properly if you're hired?

- **Using long paragraphs to describe past work experience**—Consider using a bulleted list instead. Most employers will spend less than one-minute initially reading a resume.

On the following pages you will find two resume samples of people interested in positions as pharmacy technicians.

Frank J. Rosenberg

1234 Broadway
Mytown, CA 91087
Phone and fax: (555)-559-5678
Email: Frankole89@online.com

OBJECTIVE: To work as a pharmacy technician for an employer who allows me to utilize and enhance my intelligence and strong work ethic.

EXPERIENCE

April 2001–Present
Pharmacy Technician, Mytown Pharmacy,
180 West Main Street, Mytown, CA, 91087; (555)-559-3456
Duties:
• Assist pharmacist in the filling, preparation, and delivery of medications
• Transcribe prescriptions
• Update patient profiles
• Ordere daily and weekly pharmacy inventory
• Maintain all pharmacy records

January 1999–March 2001
Data Entry Clerk, Sofitech Clinical Laboratory
1440 Ivy Road, Mytown, CA 91087; (555)-559-1040
Duties:
• Worked to recruit microbiology labs across the United States to enroll in pharmacological surveillance studies
• Entered and verified lab results, patient demographics, and other statistics for various studies involving patients in a laboratory setting

January 1998–Present
Volunteer, Dogs and Cats Shelter
RR 1, Mytown, CA 91087; (555)-559-9876
Duties:
• Interview adopters
• Write column for newsletter
• Bathe dogs

EDUCATION

• Pharmacy Technician Certificate, May 2002
  California Board of Pharmacy, 400 R Street, Suite 4070, Sacramento, CA 95814
• Associate of Arts, Humanities, and Social Sciences, May 2001
  Sofia Heights Community College, Eli Hills Campus, Mytown, CA 91087

SKILLS

Fluent in Spanish
Skilled with Windows 2000, Microsoft Excel, and Lotus
References available upon request.

Rose O'Leary

521 East Avenue
Eastville, CA
Phone and fax: (555)-559-1234
Email: roleary@online.com

OBJECTIVE: Entry-level pharmacy position that allows me to utilize my computer and customer service skills while I pursue my pharmacy technician certificate.

EDUCATION

- Associate of Science, Pharmacy Technician, May 2001
  Congers Community College, Eastville, CA
- Associate of Science, Computer Technology, December 1999
  Congers Community College, Eastville, CA

Relevant Courses:

PHARMACY TECHNICIAN	COMPUTER TECHNOLOGY
Introduction to Health Care	Lotus 1234
Pharmacology/Pharmacy Law	QBASIC
Ambulatory Pharmacy	DBASE IV
Pharmacology and Data Entry	WordPerfect
Pharmaceutical Compounding	QUICKBOOKS QUICKPAY

EXPERIENCE

June–September 2001
Pharmacy Intern, Eastville Pharmacy
180 West Main Street, Eastville, CA 91088; (555)-559-3456
Duties:

- Assisted pharmacist and pharmacy technician in all phases of pharmacy management
- Delivered prescriptions
- Interacted with customers and doctors
- Responsible for answering phones and transcribing prescriptions

September 1997–Present
Evening Manager, The Store
345 Route 66, Eastville, CA 91088, (555)-559-6543
Duties:

- Manage staff of five
- Operate cash register
- Responsible for inventory upkeep and customer satisfaction
- Assist customers

References available upon request.

THE COVER LETTER

The purpose of a cover letter is simple. It should provide the reader, your potential employer, with information on which job you are applying for, where you heard about the opening, and an overview of your qualifications.

When writing your cover letter, keep in mind that the person reading it will be busy and is likely to spend less than a minute reading your letter. It is important, therefore, to keep your letter short and succinct.

What Should You Include?

The first line of your cover letter should clearly identify the position for which you are applying. Your potential employer may have several job openings and you want to be sure that your resume is considered for the correct one. You can copy the title directly from the advertisement and state where you saw the ad. For example, your opening line may be, "Please accept my resume for Pharmacy Technician Level One advertised in the *Youngstown Morning Star* on Sunday, March 17, 2002."

Your cover letter is your opportunity to summarize your qualifications effectively. You don't need to list every course you have taken on the road to becoming a pharmacy technician. Nor do you need to list every job, internship, or volunteer position you've ever held. Limit your cover letter to statements that will make an impact such as, "I recently completed a successful pharmacy technician training program and will sit for the Pharmacy Technician Certification Exam in April."

If possible, address your cover letter to a specific person. If the advertisement does not list a name, take the time to investigate. Call the human resources department and ask for the name of the hiring manager or human resources representative. If it is company policy not to give out names, try to get a formal title and use that in place of a name. Try to avoid using *Human Resources Representative* as a name.

The following pages contain two sample cover letters.

Frank J. Rosenberg
1234 Broadway
Mytown, CA 91087
Phone and fax: (555)-559-5678
Email: Frankole89@online.com

May 11, 2002

Rennie Elberg
Program Director
Royalville Outpatient Facility
Royalville, CA 90278

Mr. Elberg:

I am writing to you in response to the advertisement in the May 10th *Royalville Times* regarding the position of pharmacy technician. I have recently gained my certification as pharmacy technician from the California Board of Pharmacy, and I am currently employed in that position in a small pharmacy in my hometown.

The experience I have gained working for my current employer is invaluable, and I am constantly searching for ways in which I can improve myself as a professional and increase my skill and knowledge level. That desire for growth is what led me to the Royalville Outpatient Facility. I am intrigued by the proposition of working for your facility because I believe that we would be an excellent fit as an employer and employee. I can offer you my incomparable work effort, my professional knowledge, and considerable skills, and you can offer me the opportunity to work in an interesting environment in which I can thrive and grow.

I would appreciate the opportunity to meet with you and discuss this further. I have attached my resume to this letter for your perusal. I appreciate your time and consideration.

Sincerely,

Frank J. Rosenberg

Frank J. Rosenberg

Enclosure.

Rose O'Leary
521 East Avenue
Eastville, CA
Phone and fax: (555)-559-1234
Email: roleary@online.com

May 12, 2002

Rory Parton
Senior Pharmacist
Little Bear Pharmacy
Little Bear, CA 91099

Dear Mr. Parton:

I am very interested in applying for the pharmacy technician position listed in the *Little Bear Register* on May 4, 2002.

As you can see from my enclosed resume, this past summer I interned for the Eastville Pharmacy. I enjoyed the work very much, and learned a tremendous amount about the responsibilities of being a pharmacy technician. In addition, I have recently decided to pursue my certification from the California Board of Pharmacy, and plan on being certified next spring. I'm an organized, detail-oriented person who gets along well with people. I was nominated for Employee of the Year twice in my tenure as the evening manager at The Store here in Eastville. I feel that these attributes, along with my work and academic experience, qualify me for the position described in your advertisement.

I would greatly appreciate the opportunity for a personal interview. You can reach me at 555-559-1234.

Thank you for your consideration.

Sincerely,

Rose O'Leary
Rose O'Leary

Enclosure.

THE INTERVIEW

This is the step in the job search processes that causes the most anxiety for job seekers. A face-to-face meeting with your potential employer gives him or her the chance to decide if you are the right person for the job, and you the chance to decide if the job is right for you. While it is normal to be nervous during an interview, there are many things you can do to calm your fears. The most worthwhile thing you can do is to gain a solid understanding of the interview process, and your role in it. By carefully reading the information below, and following the suggestions made, you will greatly improve your chances for interviewing success.

Understanding the Interview Format

When you are arranging an interview, try to find out as much as possible about the format. Who should you ask for when you arrive at the appointed time? Will you be meeting with more than one person? Where will the interview take place? Will you be expected to perform any tasks (counting tablets, measuring medication, etc.)?

The more you know about what to expect from your interview, the easier it will be to prepare and the more comfortable you will feel.

Preparing for Your Interview

Research the company before your interview and be ready to demonstrate your knowledge. If you are interviewing at a chain pharmacy, it will be easy for you to find information on the company website. The same is true of a hospital, as most have websites these days. Your library and chamber of commerce will also have information on local hospitals and may have information on local pharmacies as well. If you know other pharmacy technicians who have worked where you are interviewing, ask them if they can provide you with any insider tips.

In addition to researching the company, employ the following strategies to properly prepare for your interview and make a good first impression:

▶ Get a good night's sleep before the interview. You want to look and feel rested and be awake and alert.

▶ Before your interview, take a shower, shampoo your hair, clean your fingernails, brush your teeth, shave, and apply antiperspirant and deodorant. Your appearance is the first thing your interviewer will notice about you. First impressions count!

▶ Make sure your interview outfit is clean, free of wrinkles, and fits you perfectly. Be sure your shoes are shined and coordinate well with your outfit. You may want to consider laying out your outfit the night before your interview. If your outfit needs to go to the dry cleaner, however, take it there well in advance of your interview. You don't want to find out the day of your interview that your outfit is not clean or has shrunk and no longer fits!

▶ Make several extra copies of your resume, letters of recommendation, and a list of references. Bring these with you to your interview. Also, you should bring your daily planner, any research material, a pad, and a working pen. Write the company's name, interviewer's name, address, telephone number, and directions to the interview at the top of your pad.

▶ On the morning of your interview read your local newspaper or watch a morning news program. This way, you will be aware of the day's news events in case the interviewer wants to start off with general small talk.

▶ If you have never been to where your interview will be held, take the time to determine the best route at least a day in advance. You might even want to drive by the location to estimate the amount of time it will take you to get there, where you will park, etc.

▶ Arrive at your interview at least ten minutes early and check in. While it is okay for the interviewer to keep you waiting for a short period of time, it is *not* okay for you, the applicant, to keep your interviewer waiting for even one minute. If you have transportation troubles, and you anticipate running late, call as soon as possible to alert your interviewer.

Interview Questions

After introductions, your interviewer will ask you several questions. The exact questions will depend on the interviewer's personal style but there are fairly standard questions that you can expect to be asked in one form or another. Since pharmacy technicians have specific skill-sets, you should anticipate detailed questions about your skills and the experience you have using them.

As part of your job interview preparation, you can think about the types of questions the interviewer will ask and how you will answer them. Take the time to develop thoughtful, complete, and intelligent answers. You will benefit even more from actual practice answering interview questions out loud. Stage a mock interview with someone who will evaluate your responses honestly.

Most of the questions you will be asked will be pretty obvious, but be prepared for an interviewer to ask you a few that are unexpected. By doing this, the interviewer will be able to see how you react and how well you think on your feet.

The following are common interview questions and suggestions on how you can best answer them:

- ▶ What can you tell me about yourself?
- ▶ Why have you chosen to pursue a career as a pharmacy technician?
- ▶ What are your career objectives?
- ▶ What do you expect to be doing in five years?
- ▶ What are your long-term goals?
- ▶ Tell me about your training program.
- ▶ What courses interested you the most? The least?
- ▶ What is your previous work experience?
- ▶ What jobs have you enjoyed the most? The least? Why?
- ▶ What do you consider to be your major strengths and weaknesses?
- ▶ In your personal or professional life, what has been your greatest failure? What did you learn from that experience?
- ▶ If you could have the perfect position, what would it be?
- ▶ Why should we hire you?
- ▶ In what ways do you think you can make a contribution to our pharmacy?

▶ Why do you think you're the most qualified person to fill this job?

▶ What two or three accomplishments have given you the most satisfaction?

▶ What have you done to show initiative and willingness to work?

▶ Do you subscribe to trade journals or magazines? If so, which ones?

▶ What qualifications do you have that make you feel you will be successful in this field?

▶ What else can you tell me about yourself that isn't listed in your resume?

Guidelines for Answering Questions

Your interviewer will be evaluating you on how you answer his or her questions. Keep the following points in mind:

▶ Speak clearly, using complete sentences and proper English. "Yeah," is never an acceptable answer to an interview question.

▶ Don't be evasive, especially if you're asked about any negative aspects of your employment history.

▶ Don't imply that a question is "stupid" or "silly."

▶ Always tell the truth—don't stretch it.

▶ Be prepared to answer the same questions multiple times. Make sure your answers are consistent, and never reply, "You already asked me that."

▶ Never apologize for negative information regarding your past.

▶ Avoid talking down to an interviewer, or making them feel less intelligent than you are.

Interviewing Your Interviewer

An interview works two ways: An employer wants to find out about you, and you should want to find out about them. After all, you want to feel confident that you have chosen the right place to work. Frequently, toward the close of the interview, the interviewer will provide the opportunity to ask questions. If you don't ask any questions, your interviewer may think you are not interested in the position. Prepare your questions in advance, and ask the most important questions first, in case there is not enough time to ask all of them. This is your chance to set yourself apart from the competition; don't ask questions that might show a lack of research. Some examples of questions you might want to ask are:

▶ What would my typical day consist of?
▶ What would my level of responsibility be?
▶ What are the work hours?
▶ Do pharmacy technicians attend educational seminars?
▶ Will there be opportunities for hands-on training?
▶ What other help can you offer as I move up and become more experienced?
▶ Are health benefits offered?
▶ Is there a 401(k) or some other form of employee savings plan?
▶ Is there a training or procedures manual in which my specific duties or responsibilities are spelled out?

At the Interview

You've prepared. You're confident in your skills and abilities. You're wearing your best outfit and you feel rested and ready to make a good impression. Follow these tactics and you will be sure to do just that.

▶ From the moment you arrive at your interview location, be in interview mode. Act professionally and be polite to everyone you meet—including secretaries, receptionists, cashiers, and other technicians.
▶ When you are introduced to your interviewer, stand up, smile, make direct eye contact, and shake hands. Refer to your interviewer formally, as Mr./Ms./Dr. (insert last name).
▶ Throughout your interview, sit up straight. Listen carefully to each question and take a moment or two to formulate your answers, and then answer in complete sentences.

▶ Be aware of your body language. Crossing your arms in front of your chest may be perceived as defiant by an interviewer. Looking away from your interviewer when being asked a question could be perceived as disinterest. Keep your body language in check and your interviewer will have a better assessment of you.

▶ During the later part of your interview, make a point to ask for the job you're applying for. Explain exactly why you want the job, what you can offer, and why you're the best candidate for the position.

Communicate Your Communication Skills

Don't be so intent on selling yourself that you fail to show your true communication skills. Take the time to listen when your interviewer is explaining the position, job responsibilities, and work environment. Ask thoughtful questions when appropriate, but don't interrupt your interviewer. Take your time in replying to questions. A slow, thoughtful response is best. Smile—and breathe. Show your interviewer that you have the communication and people skills required for pharmacy technicians.

FOLLOW-UP

After the interview, follow up with a thank-you note to the interviewer. This shows the interviewer that you are serious about the position and helps them to remember you better. Here are some tips for following up:

▶ Have plenty of paper and stamps available. A thank-you note is most effective when it is written on the same day as your interview and mailed right away. You can use the same paper as you use for your cover letters and resumes, or use note cards specifically for thank-you notes.

▶ Send a separate note to each person who interviewed you, and make each note personal. Refer to something that happened or that you discussed during the interview.

▶ Check your note for spelling and grammatical errors. You are trying to reinforce the impression that you are the right candidate for the job.

Many job seekers fail to send out thank-you notes after interviews. Apparently, they believe that the interviewer is simply doing his or her job. This is a mistake that you should not make.

Sending a personal and considerate note after an interview is extremely beneficial. It will keep your name in the forefront of your potential employer's mind. It will show that you have good follow-up skills and that you're truly interested in the position. And, if the other candidates don't show their gratitude with a thank-you note, you will really stand out from the competition.

Be sure to keep your message brief and to the point. After thanking your interviewer for his or her time, highlight the important details discussed in your interview. You want your interviewer to remember you in a positive way. Summarize the reasons why you are the right candidate for the position and reaffirm your interest in the position. Invite further contact with a closing line such as "I look forward to hearing from you soon."

Do not discuss salary, benefits, work schedule, start dates or other concerns. Those issues should only be discussed after you have a job offer.

Fast Facts

According to the *Occupational Outlook Handbook*, employers prefer pharmacy technician applicants with strong customer service and communication skills and experience managing inventories, counting, measuring, and using a computer. They also want technicians who have strong spelling and reading skills.

Source: United States Department of Labor, Occupational Outlook Handbook

THE JOB OFFER

When the phone rings and you are offered the job you were hoping for, you will undoubtedly be excited. Enthusiasm is terrific, but don't let it get in the way of making sure you are getting the best offer. If you haven't already addressed compensation issues, do so before accepting the job. Find out exactly how you will be paid, how often, and whether or not you will be eligible for overtime.

The Importance of Benefits

Be sure to ask your prospective employer about the benefits program. Specifically, query them about the following:

- ▶ **Health Insurance**—Ask if health insurance is employee-paid, company-paid or a combination of the two.
- ▶ **Company-funded profit sharing**—Many pharmacies offer some type of profit sharing, to which both the employer and employee contribute. Employees become fully vested in the plan after a period of years.
- ▶ **401(k) plans**—As with profit sharing, both parties kick in contributions to this plan. However, you can't withdraw the money before age $59\frac{1}{2}$ without a steep penalty, making this an ideal retirement account.
- ▶ **Paid vacations**—An obvious perk!
- ▶ **Training programs and education**—Ask whether the pharmacy will pay for any advanced classes or seminars you'd like to take.

LAST THOUGHTS ON INTERVIEWING

There are two more important things to keep in mind while going through interviews. Both will help you to keep not only your interview, but the whole job search process, in perspective. The first is that even if you apply and interview for a job, you don't have to take it. The other is that good interviewers try to sell you on coming to work for them. Understanding that you are not required to take a job just because it's offered makes the interview seem less like a life-or-death situation and more like an opportunity to get to know at least one person in the pharmacy profession. You will feel a greater sense of confidence and ease when you keep this in mind. Remember, the pharmacy technician position you're interviewing for isn't the only one available, so if it feels like a bad fit for you, or for them, move on.

Realizing that interviewers are selling you on coming to work for them is helpful, too. A good interviewer has one goal in mind—finding a good person to fill the job opening. They already think you're a possibility, which is why you were invited to interview. Once you're there, it's the interviewer's job to convince you that you would be very happy working at this particular establishment. Evaluate the information you're given about the work environment; does it fit with what you see and have heard about the pharmacy? Be attuned to the tactics of the interviewer.

Finally, there will be an end to the job search process. You will be offered a position that meets your wants and needs, and you will accept it. Chapter 6 details what happens after you begin work, helping you to maximize your potential for success in your new career.

THE INSIDE TRACK

Who: Dora Henderson
What: CPhT
Where: Greeley, Colorado

I work in a hospital-based outpatient infusion clinic. I'm sort of a hybrid—I know a lot about insurances and obtaining authorizations for treatment/drugs, but I also spend a great deal of my day entering orders and mixing sterile preparations—IVs, epidurals, intrathecals and TPNs. I have an Associates of Arts degree and was certified as CPhT in 1998. I love my job, and was very fortunate in finding it—when the infusion clinic opened, the pharmacist in charge more or less drafted me for the job. I have had the opportunity to create my dream job. If I want to try something new, or expand my duties or knowledge I pretty much develop my own game plan—with my director's blessing. My current position was the first of its kind in our hospital, so there were no set qualifications. . . . I sort of made things up as I went along shaping my job description to meet the needs of the department. In addition, I was the first CPhT at our facility.

Like many other technicians, I originally joined the profession with the idea in the back of my mind that I would become a pharmacist. However, since the development of national certification, I have become a very vocal proponent of the "tech movement." I believe we are on the verge of a major shift in the way techs are viewed and used. More and more states are recognizing the CPhT status. I believe the Pharmacy Technician Certification Board (PTCB) needs to raise the bar so to speak—restricting those who can sit for the exam to only those who are in, or have graduated from, a National Association Board of Pharmacy-approved tech training program, or are currently employed (in a technician capacity) at a pharmacy. I also believe the written test should be followed by a day of practical exams.

Throughout my career, I've met some incredible people who have literally changed my life. I wouldn't be as active and outspoken about techs if it weren't for the pharmacists I have worked with, and the patients I have encountered. Each day is special and there is always something to be learned, experienced, or shared. I also enjoy the sense of "family" we have at work.

A good work ethic is the most important quality for pharmacy technicians. Critical thinking skills, flexibility, creativity, tons of compassion, a desire to strive for excellence, and to never stop learning are all essential. Self-respect and respect of patients/ customers and coworkers are also important. If you truly believe you have these skills, my advice for you is to go for it!

CHAPTER six

HOW TO SUCCEED ONCE YOU'VE LANDED THE JOB

YOUR FIRST JOB should be one that you will thoroughly enjoy and that will lead you toward future career growth. The skills and habits you develop on your own are part of the foundation that will determine the level of success you will have in your career. This chapter provides tips on forging positive relationships with your boss and coworkers, and advice on fitting into the work culture. You will also learn about paying your dues and moving up, managing your time, and making your mark while on the job.

MANAGING WORK RELATIONSHIPS—BASIC RULES

You may not have been aware of it, but you began establishing your professional reputation while you were in your training program. Did you show up to your classes on time? Good—you have a reputation for being responsible. Did you spearhead your school's participation in a local Komen Race for the Cure for breast cancer fundraising? Excellent—you have a reputation for doing more than you have to do. You built on that reputation when you began applying for jobs and participating in job interviews. Your professional reputation is what people think of you in terms of your personality, competence, and attitude. This perception contributes greatly to what

Success Strategy

Seize every opportunity to learn something new about the pharmacy world. Pharmacy magazines are excellent resources and are filled with articles that relate to the work of pharmacy technicians. For example, recent issues of pharmacy magazines contained articles on topics such as pill splitting, tracking "missing" medications in hospitals, and Oxycontin abuse. A good magazine to subscribe to is *Today's Technician*, published by the National Pharmacy Technicians Association

coworkers, pharmacists, patients, and anyone else you come into professional contact with might say or think about you when you are not around.

No matter what type of practice setting you choose, part of your success will depend on the on-the-job relationships you develop and cultivate. This refers to how you get along with others, both those you work with and the patients or customers you serve. Making a conscious effort to respect others and ensuring that you're a team player while on the job will help your career immensely.

When it comes to building and maintaining professional relationships, some basic rules apply to any workplace.

1. **Sometimes peace is better than justice.**

You may be sure you are right about a specific situation. Unfortunately, your coworkers or supervising pharmacist may disagree with you. This is a common occurrence in the workplace, especially in a pharmacy when you are just starting out. Sometimes it will be appropriate to assert your position and convince others to trust your judgment. Your previous track record and reputation will go a long way in helping people to trust your opinions, ideas, and decisions. Just be sure to choose your battles wisely. For instance, go ahead and argue your position if you can prevent a catastrophe. Who can forget young George Bailey saving Mr. Gower from sending poison to his patient in *It's a Wonderful Life*? Let your recommendation(s) be known, but do not argue your point relentlessly. Sometimes you will be right and people will not listen to you. Always be open to compromise and be willing to listen to and consider the options and ideas of others. Remember, the pharmacist has training that you do not have. You need to respect and learn from that.

2. **Don't burn bridges.**

Think of your career as a long and winding path on which you travel from experience to experience. The people with whom you interact throughout your career are the bridges connecting various portions of your path. You never know how many times you will come upon the same bridge during your journey. If you burn it in a fit of self-righteousness, an entire portion of your potential path could be closed to you.

Keep in mind that your professional reputation will follow you throughout your career. It takes years to build a positive reputation, but only one mistake could destroy it. If you wind up acting unprofessionally toward someone, even if you don't ever have contact with that person again, he or she will have contact with many other people and possibly describe you as hard-to-work-with or downright rude. Your work reputation is very important; don't tarnish it by burning your bridges.

3. **Keep work and your social life separate.**

While it's important to be friendly and form positive relationships with the people you work with, beware of becoming too chummy. Personal relationships can wreak havoc in the workplace, especially if those relationships turn sour. Consider that you might have to rate a friend's job performance, or fire someone you hang out with. If you become friends with a coworker, you may want to have a conversation with him or her to outline the crossover between your friendship and work relationship. Some people refuse to discuss work issues outside of the workplace. Setting boundaries will help your relationship succeed in the long term.

Managing Your Relationship with Your Boss

A boss is part teacher and part supervisor, and often (but not always) a registered pharmacist. He or she expects you to succeed and will do everything within reason to ensure that you do, but your success ultimately depends on you. Use your insight to study your boss. Pay attention to what she says; watch her manner. It's important that you understand her professional values so you can meet performance expectations.

It's also very important to keep the communication lines open. Talk to your boss about her management style and adjust your expectations to work within that style. For instance, your first boss might like to be hands-on and help you troubleshoot problems. She might want to talk to you at least once a day to hear about your activities. You need to understand that this boss wants to empower you through a mentoring/teaching style.

On the other hand, your second boss might want you to call him only if you have a problem. You need to understand that this boss wants to empower you through a hands-off style that lets you find your own solutions. Both bosses may be good managers; they simply have different styles. Understand the value of each style and get the most from it.

Also talk to your boss about *your* career goals. Set goals for six months, one year, three years, and five years. Based on your discussions, you and your boss can create strategies to lead you toward your goals. For example, if you are a people person and an organizer, you might want to move toward a management position and set relevant goals. No matter what you are interested in, make a plan, share it with your boss, and get a few steps closer to achieving your goals.

Success Strategy

If you don't understand something, ask. Don't assume you will be able to figure out what the pharmacist is asking you to do unless you're absolutely sure you will be able to. It's always best to ask a simple clarifying question rather than making a potentially deadly mistake. It is absolutely critical that you remember that your precision can sometimes mean the difference between life and death.

Dealing with a Difficult Boss

If you're in a situation where you simply don't see eye-to-eye with your boss, you have several options. You can do nothing, live with the situation, hope that it doesn't get worse, and not let your relationship with your boss impact you emotionally. Or, you can quit your job and seek employment elsewhere. Either of these might appear to be the easiest solution to your problem, but neither will most likely lead to long-term career fulfillment.

Another option is to carefully evaluate your situation and choose to alter *your* attitude and behavior, and to do whatever it takes to develop a relationship with your boss that evolves around mutual respect. Developing this type of professional relationship doesn't mean you will become best friends with your boss, but it does mean that you should find a way to work together so that you're both happy and productive.

Dealing with a difficult boss can be extremely hard to handle. One of the worst situations is when a boss is unethical in the way he performs his job. In this case, be sure that you document all of your work and accomplishments. When dealing directly with your boss, make sure that other people are present, and never agree to do anything that might jeopardize your reputation or job. If your boss' actions are illegal or unethical, it might be necessary to take measures to protect yourself and your career.

On the other hand, having an occasional disagreement with a superior is normal. If your life is being compromised by the actions of a mean or difficult boss, it's up to you to take action and find a solution with which you can be happy.

Success Strategy

October is "National Talk about Prescriptions Month." Why not talk to your pharmacist about honoring the month by arranging a community open house at your pharmacy? During the month, encourage members of the pharmacy team to spend extra time discussing prescriptions with patients.

Managing Relationships with Your Coworkers

You will meet many people in the course of your career. Some you will admire; some you will find barely tolerable. For your personal development, you need to find a way to work well with everyone—even if they're not your best friends. Acknowledging and accepting someone else's talents and expertise is very different from being their close friend, yet in the workplace, maintaining professional respect for the people you work with will allow everyone to be more productive and successful.

The following are some fundamental rules for fostering positive working relationships with your peers:

▶ **Don't gossip about your supervising pharmacist, manager, fellow technicians, or anyone else.** Gossip hurts the person being talked about, will inevitably come back to haunt you, and can make you look like you don't have enough to do.

▶ **Foster sharing relationships instead of competitive relationships.** If you read an interesting article in a pharmacy magazine, or find a new source for Continuing Education courses, share the information with the other technicians. A group of people who help each other develop professionally will shine as a team and as individuals. On the other hand, if you jockey for position and compete over everything, you will miss out on the wealth that you could learn from more experienced technicians (and will have to work in a competitive, strained environment).

▶ **Don't become a loner, only looking out for you.** When it comes time for employee evaluations or when you're being considered for a raise, you want to be thought of as a hard working, sincere, honest, team player who does his or her best work in the interest of the pharmacy as a whole.

Your workplace peers can be the greatest pleasure of your job—or your biggest pain. As with your boss, it's best to put your observational skills to the test. If you do, you will soon identify the hardest workers, the chronic complainers, and the clock-watchers.

It's hard to know where to draw the line with colleagues, particularly if you're fond of them all. A good rule of thumb to remember is: They're your coworkers, not your family. Don't get overly involved in their lives. Remember the purpose of your job—to help you develop your career.

Some other tips:

▶ **Always be friendly and professional.** If you're having a bad day (the car broke down, the baby is sick, your tax return was smaller than expected), try to push that aside. Practice treating your coworkers the same way you treat your patients.

▶ **Don't get involved in disputes.** Unless you witness something un-ethical on the job—and think perhaps the supervising pharmacist or manager should be made aware of it—keep quiet. It's a no-win situation otherwise.

▶ **Solve your own conflicts.** Don't get your boss involved unless the situation is so bad that you want to leave your job and you believe he can do something about the problem. Dragging him into personality disputes will only make him think less of you as a technician.

▶ **Don't let praise go to your head**—and don't take criticism to heart.

▶ **Always behave responsibly.** Your supervisor should outline what will and will not be tolerated on the job, and you need to abide by her outline. For example, if you are not allowed to make personal calls during work hours, don't make them.

▶ **Be approachable.** Have lunch with the group; don't hide in the back room. You want to feel comfortable with your coworkers and you want them to feel comfortable with you. You can learn a lot from each other's experiences.

▶ **Treat everyone equally.** You will always have favorite coworkers, and others you might half-wish not to have. As a responsible person, however, you should treat even the people you dislike in a fair manner.

Know Your Rights

Pregnancy discrimination laws prevent employers from penalizing you because of pregnancy, including loss of pay or job benefits, or even reassigning you to other positions under the pretext of protecting your pregnancy. If you experience a job loss, loss in pay, or loss of position in a company, consult a lawyer immediately. Keep in mind that the Federal Family and Medical Leave Act (FMLA) grants a cumulative 12 weeks of leave in a 12-month period. However, you may be entitled to more leave under state laws or your company plan.

MANAGING YOUR TIME

You will most likely find that the workplace environment is more hectic than school was, so you will need to manage your time effectively to make the most of your workweek. Here are some tips for juggling your tasks and managing your time.

1. **Know the requirements of your job and what your boss expects of you.** Define your role and know what is expected of you on a daily basis.

2. **Don't get trapped by interruptions and time wasters.** Every job is subject to time wasters. If you work with a social, chatty person, don't let yourself be distracted or interrupted.

3. **Keep a day planner.** Identify one place where you write everything down, whether it is a formal day planner or a spiral notebook. Are you always running late for appointments? Do the items on your daily to-do list never seem to get done fast enough? Do you feel that you don't have any spare time to learn and develop new skills? If there is never enough time in your day to meet your personal and professional obligations, you could be lacking important time management skills.

If you find that this is an area in which you could improve, begin to do so immediately. Learning time management skills won't add more hours to the work day, but it will allow you to use all of your time more productively, reduce the stress in your life, better focus on what's important, and ultimately get more done, faster. If you've decided to use a time management tool such as a computer program or personal digital assistant, spend the time necessary to learn how to use it properly. These tools are only as effective as their user, and although it may take a large time investment to get started, it will be well worth it.

Next, over the course of several days, analyze how you spend every minute of your day. Determine what takes up the majority of your time, but diminishes your productivity. Perhaps you experience countless interruptions from coworkers, you make long telephone calls, you don't have well-defined priorities, your work area is messy and disorganized, or you have too much to do and become overwhelmed. As you examine how you spend your day, pinpoint the biggest time wasters that are keeping you from getting your most important work done.

Take major projects, goals, and objectives and divide them into smaller, more manageable tasks. You will need to incorporate your to-do list into your daily planner, allowing you to schedule your time. Make sure you attempt to complete your high-priority items and tasks early in the day, giving those items your full attention. Also, make sure you list all of your pre-scheduled appointments in your daily schedule, allowing ample time to get to and from the appointments and, if necessary, prepare for them in advance.

Once you commit to using a time management tool, it's important to remain disciplined, using it continuously until it becomes second nature. Initially, you may have to spend up to 30 minutes per day planning your time and creating your to-do list, but ultimately, you will begin saving up to several hours per day. Learning to better manage your time will boost your productivity, which will ultimately make you more valuable to your employer, putting you in a better position to receive a raise or promotion.

MANAGING LIFE AND A JOB

When you are at work every day all week long, it becomes difficult to get your *life tasks* done. When you have a family, and you're juggling the needs and schedules of a number of people, it can be even more difficult. Just as with your job, the key to getting everything done (with spare time to relax!) is organization. Here are some tips to help you integrate your job with your life.

▶ **Make "to-do" lists and prioritize the tasks you need to accomplish.** Keep a list of things you need to do, buy, return, pick up, and drop off. A day planner is the best place to keep such a list. If you don't have a day planner, carry a notebook with you from home to work and back again. Organize your list according to places you will stop. Keep grocery items on one list, dry cleaning on another, etc. Cross things off the lists when you have finished them so you can see what you have to do at a glance.

▶ **Use your lunch hour to run errands at least once a week.** Identify resources that are close to your work for things you can do during your lunch hour—doctor, dentist, dry cleaner, shoe repair, hardware store, and so on.

▶ **Use the commute between home and work for larger errands.** This is the perfect time to get that oil change or to stop at the grocery store.

Money Saving Tips

Your first job means money in your pocket, ready to be spent. Before you rush out to spend what you have not yet earned, take a moment to consider that true maturity comes from knowing how to spend wisely and save wisely. Here some tips to help you start saving money:

- Make your own coffee in the morning rather than stopping at the local coffee shop, and eat breakfast at home.
- Bring your lunch.
- When grocery shopping, make a list beforehand and stick to it. If you have a plan going in, you will be less likely to purchase impulse (and often expensive) items.
- If you are eligible to participate in a 401(k) plan, join up as soon as possible and put in as much of your salary as you can. You will save in taxes immediately and you will be building for your retirement.
- Find out if your pharmacy offers direct deposit of paychecks. If it does, choose to have either a percent or set amount ($25 per paycheck, for example) deposited into your savings account.
- Make a budget with short-term and long-term saving goals.
- Pay off your debt! Start with lenders that charge the highest interest (department store credit cards are notorious for their high interest rates) and work your way down to the lowest interest.

SURVIVING YOUR FIRST WEEKS AT A NEW JOB

For many job seekers, the stress involved with finding new job opportunities, sending out resumes, participating in interviews and dealing with all of the other hassles involved with finding employment can be emotionally draining. Thus, it makes perfect sense that most people experience a huge sense of relief once they're actually offered a new job, conduct a successful salary negotiation, and then accept a new position.

The problem is, as soon as some people show up for their first day of work, the stress associated with beginning a new job kicks in, which could make the first few weeks at a new job unpleasant. Stepping into a new job situation can be difficult. It often involves a major change in your daily routine, getting to know an entirely new group of people, and learning the policies and procedures of your new employer.

You also need to learn about the underlying politics that play a major role in any work environment, and determine exactly what is expected of you in terms of job performance. It's necessary to determine exactly how you fit in the operation of the pharmacy and be willing to adapt your work habits to meet the needs of your employer.

Hopefully, before accepting your job, you did research to learn about the pharmacy and what you'd be doing there, so you're confident you've found the right job for you. If you go into a new job knowing there's a good chance you're going to enjoy it, the stress associated with starting the job will be greatly diminished, since much of the stress you'd typically feel would be in anticipation of entering into an unknown situation.

Adapting to a new work situation happens instantaneously for some, but for others could take up to three or four weeks. As a new pharmacy technician, you will be constantly learning, so there will be adjustments for you to make throughout your first year. During this time, be open-minded and try to maintain a positive attitude, no matter how unhappy or stressed out you are. Until some time has passed, it's difficult to tell if you've simply accepted the wrong job, or if you're experiencing the new job acclimation process, which is normal. Unless you're absolutely sure you've made the wrong job decision by accepting your job after a week or two, stick it out for at least a month before making the decision to quit if you're still unhappy.

During your first few weeks at a new job, there are several things you can do to help yourself and your coworkers become more comfortable. First, instead of confronting people who may give you a difficult time, try to fit in right from the start by being friendly toward everyone. Also, ask questions to demonstrate a desire to learn how things are done, and whenever possible, attempt to strike up non-work-related conversations, especially during lunch or break periods. This will help you get to know the people you're working with on a personal level.

Always think of a new job as providing a new set of exciting opportunities and a chance to start fresh. By taking control of your life, you can seek out and pursue those opportunities that will lead to career advancement and happiness. You must, however, face these opportunities with the proper mindset and be willing to work hard for what you want. Never allow the fear of failing to hold you back as you begin to take advantage of the opportunities your new job has to offer.

If you begin your new job determined to be open minded, professional, friendly, persistent and flexible, chances are you will adapt quickly and soon be accepted by your new coworkers.

PROMOTING YOURSELF

There are a number of other things you can do to keep your career moving in a positive direction. You can't wait for opportunities to land in your lap; rather, you need to be proactive by promoting yourself. Then, you will create opportunity for yourself. Keeping track of what you do and when you do it will create a permanent record of your accomplishments—something you will want to have as verification if your work is ever called into question, or remembered incorrectly. Finally, by handling any criticism professionally, remaining calm, listening to what is said, and offering to make changes, you will come out on top even in the stickiest of situations. Next, ways of promoting yourself will be discussed in greater detail.

Taking Control of Your Duties and Tasks

You may find yourself working for a pharmacist or pharmacists who still aren't sure what a pharmacy technician can do. They might, out of ignorance, think of you as a clerk, only able to do a very limited number of things, such as ring up customers or answer the telephone. They may not realize that you are capable of filling prescriptions, or maintaining equipment. You need to prove your knowledge and competency to the pharmacists. When you begin your job, make sure all of the pharmacists with whom you will be working know the level of training you have completed. If you are certified, or are studying to take the exam, let them know.

If you find that you are being asked to perform only clerical duties, live with it for a few weeks until you feel completely comfortable with the work environment and are sure that you have learned the systems at your place of employment. Your supervising pharmacist may be reluctant to give you tasks he knows you can handle until he is convinced that you have mastered all of the basics of the practice setting. For example, he may want to be sure that you are adept at using the cash register and the patient database before moving you on to starting to fill prescriptions. If that is the case, you will see that you are being directed toward more advanced tasks within a few weeks to two months.

If your duties do not change, and you are still relegated only to the cash register after two months, you need to speak up. Ask the pharmacist if you can speak to her to talk about how you are progressing on the job. Then, in a non-accusatory tone and manner, tell her that you are disappointed that your duties and responsibilities are not in-line with your capabilities. Give her specific examples of the work you have been doing and then contrast that with specific examples of the work you believe you could do, and do well.

When you are given the opportunity to perform the duties for which you were hired, do everything you can to ensure you perform them well. Take the extra steps to prove that you are a valuable member of the pharmacy team.

Building on Your Reputation

No matter how well you work with others and how organized you are, in the end you will be judged by how well you perform your duties. You want to develop a reputation as someone who does his or her job well, on time, and in a consistent manner. To accomplish this, whenever someone gives you a task, make sure you know exactly what is expected of you.

Handling Criticism

At some point in your career, it is likely that you will receive criticism about your job performance. You may be a model technician, but somewhere down the road you will either work with a difficult pharmacist or other supervisor, or you will be doing something that is genuinely worthy of criticism. When you do receive criticism, you need to do three things. The first is to remain calm. You need to hear what is being said, and that is nearly impossible when you're upset. Listen and understand what is being said without trying to defend yourself or correcting the person who's critiquing your work.

Second, ask for clarification and concrete help to rectify the situation. If you've been told that you need to be more on top of things, find out exactly what the problem is. Do you need to be more on top of inventory? Do you need to answer the phone on fewer rings? Are you making errors on your prescription labels that the pharmacist repeatedly has to fix? These are quite different issues. You need to discover what the problem is and learn how to make it right.

Third, follow any advice given, and ask the person who's critiquing you for help in the future. By keeping calm, and responding in a non-defensive, professional manner, you can turn a negative critique into an opportunity for positive growth and change.

HELPFUL RESOURCES

There is a wide range of information and resources available to help you succeed in your career as a pharmacy technician. Books, magazines, and websites are obvious resources. Your supervising pharmacist, fellow pharmacy technicians, and other coworkers are resources as well. Take advantage of every opportunity to build your knowledge base.

Throughout this book, you have been provided with websites to assist in your training, job search, and career development. Once you are on the job, these sites will continue to be of value to you. Bookmark all pharmacy and healthcare-related sites and visit them often.

In addition to the resources you've already read about so far, you can find a comprehensive list of websites and publications in Appendix B, in the back of this book.

COLLECTING INFORMATION

When you read an article that directly pertains to the work you do on a day-to-day basis, or come across tips that could enhance your efficacy, you should keep the information handy. One way to do so is with your day planner or a separate notebook. If you choose to collect important information in your day planner, be sure that you designate a section specifically for that use. In your planner or notebook, make notes and insert articles or other important information. Then, carry the notebook with you to work every day and refer to it when necessary. You will probably be surprised how often you find yourself doing so.

Two examples of information that will be helpful in your daily work life are common conversions and the top 200 prescriptions. They are listed on the following pages to help you get started collecting information.

COMMON CONVERSIONS

You will find that certain doctors will write out prescriptions differently than others. For example, some will write a prescription for 25 ug of a drug while others may write 0.025 mg. You need to be aware that these amounts are the same. Here are some common conversions:

1000 ug (micrograms) = 1 mg (milligram)
1000 mg (milligrams) = 1 g (gram)
1 cc (cubic centimeter) = 1 ml (milliliter)
5 ml (milliliter) is approximately 1 teaspoon
15 ml (milliliter) is approximately 1 tablespoon
30 ml (milliliter) is approximately 1 oz (ounce)
480 ml (milliliter) is approximately 1 pint
20 drops is approximately 1 ml (milliliter)
30 g (gram) is approximately 1 oz (ounce)

Top 200 Prescriptions for 2000 by Number of U.S. Prescriptions Dispensed

Brand Name	Manufacturer	Generic Name
Hydrocodone w/APAP	Various	Hydrocodone w/APAP
Lipitor	Parke-Davis	Atorvastatin
Premarin	Wyeth-Ayerst	Conjugated Estrogens
Synthroid	Knoll	Levothyroxine
Atenolol	Various	Atenolol
Furosemide (oral)	Various	Furosemide
Prilosec	Astra	Omeprazole
Albuterol	Various	Albuterol
Norvasc	Pfizer	Amlodipine
Alprazolam	Various	Alprazolam
Propoxyphene N/APAP	Various	Propoxyphene N/APAP
Glucophage	B-M Squibb	Metformin
Cephalexin	Various	Cephalexin
Amoxicillin	Various	Amoxicillin
Claritin	Schering	Loratadine
Trimox	Apothecon	Amoxicillin
Hydrochlorothiazide	Various	Hydrochlorothiazide
Zoloft	Pfizer	Sertraline
Zithromax (Z-Pack)	Pfizer	Azithromycin
Prozac	Lilly	Fluoxetine
Ibuprofen	Various	Ibuprofen
Paxil	SK Beecham	Paroxetine
Triamterene/HCTZ	Various	Triamterene/HCTZ
Celebrex	Searle	Celecoxib
Acetaminophen/Codeine	Various	Acetaminophen/Codeine
Prevacid	Tap Pharm	Lansoprazole
Zestril	Zeneca	Lisinopril
Augmentin	SK Beecham	Amoxicillin/Clavulanate
Prempro	Wyeth-Ayerst	Conj. Estrogens/ Medroxyprogesterone
Prednisone (oral)	Various	Prednisone
Zocor	Merck	Simvastatin

Brand Name	Manufacturer	Generic Name
Vioxx	Merck	Rofecoxib
Ortho Tri-Cyclen	Ortho Pharm	Norgestimate/Ethinyl Estradiol
Lorazepam	Various	Lorazepam
Trimethoprim/Sulfa	Various	Trimeth/Sulfameth
Lanoxin	Glaxo Wellcome	Digoxin
Metoprolol Tartrate	Various	Metoprolol
Amitriptyline	Various	Amitriptyline
Ranitidine	Various	Ranitidine
Levoxyl	Jones Medical Ind	Levothyroxine
Allegra	Hoech Mar R	Fexofenadine
Amoxil	SK Beecham	Amoxicillin
Cipro	Bayer Pharm	Ciprofloxacin
Ambien	Searle	Zolpidem
Zyrtec	Pfizer	Cetirizine
Naproxen	Various	Naproxen
Coumadin	Dupont	Warfarin
Accupril	Parke-Davis	Quinapril
Pravachol	B-M Squibb	Pravastatin
Viagra	Pfizer	Sildenafil Citrate
Glyburide	Various	Glyburide
Cyclobenzaprine	Various	Cyclobenzaprine
Toprol-XL	Astra	Metoprolol
Ultram	McNeil	Tramadol
Glucotrol-XL	Pfizer	Glipizide
Flonase	Glaxo Wellcome	Fluticasone
Verapamil SR	Various	Verapamil
Trazodone	Various	Trazodone
Prinivil	Merck	Lisinopril
Diazepam	Mylan	Diazepam
Clonazepam	Various	Clonazepam
Celexa	Forest Pharm	Citalopram
Neurontin	Parke-Davis	Gabapentin
Vasotec	Merck	Enalapril
Medroxyprogesterone	Various	Medroxyprogesterone
K-Dur	Key Pharm	Potassium Chloride

Brand Name	Manufacturer	Generic Name
Fosamax	Merck	Alendronate
Wellbutrin SR	Glaxo Well	Bupropion HCL
Carisoprodol	Various	Carisoprodol
Diflucan	Pfizer	Fluconazole
Levaquin	McNeil	Levofloxacin
Potassium Chloride	Various	Potassium Chloride
Doxycycline	Various	Doxycycline
Lotensin	Novartis	Benazepril
Flovent	Glaxo Wellcome	Fluticasone Propionate
Albuterol (nebulized)	Various	Albuterol
Singulair	Schein	Montelukast
Effexor XR	Wyeth-Ayerst	Venlafaxine
Cardura	Pfizer	Doxazosin
Biaxin	Abbott	Clarithromycin
Depakote	Abbott	Divalproex
Allopurinol	Various	Allopurinol
Isosorbide Mononitrate	Various	Isosorbide Mononitrate S.A.
Zithromax (susp)	Pfizer	Azithromycin
Humulin N	Lilly	Human Insulin NPH
Methylprednisolone	Various	Methylprednisolone
Estradiol	Various	Estradiol
Nasonex	Schering	Mometasone
Veetids	Apothecon	Penicillin VK
Cozaar	Merck	Losartan
Claritin D 12HR	Schering	Loratidine/Pseudoephedrine
Clonidine	Various	Clonidine
Warfarin	Various	Warfarin
Claritin D 24HR	Schering	Loratidine/Pseudoephedrine
Xalatan	Pharmacia/Upjohn	Latanoprost
Adderall	Shire Rchwd	Amphetamine Mixed Salts
Serevent	Glaxo Wellcome	Salmeterol
Monopril	B-M Squibb	Fosinopril
Temazepam	Various	Temazepam
Risperdal	Janssen	Risperidone
Hydroxyzine	Various	Hydroxyzine

Brand Name	Manufacturer	Generic Name
Meclizine	Various	Meclizine
Cartia XT	Andrx	Diltiazem
Pepcid	Merck	Famotidine
Plavix	Sanofi	Clopidogrel
Allegra-D	Hoech Mar R	Fexofenadine/Pseudoephedrine
Triphasil	Wyeth-Ayerst	Norgestrel/Ethinyl Estradiol
Ortho-Novum 7/7/7	Ortho Pharm	Norethindrone/Ethinyl Estradiol
Cefzil	B-M Squibb	Cefprozil
Ziac	Lederle	Bisoprolol/HCTZ
Adalat CC	Bayer Pharm	Nifedipine
Dilantin	Parke-Davis	Phenytoin
Folic Acid	Various	Folic Acid
Penicillin VK	Various	Penicillin VK
Metronidazole	Various	Metronidazole
Diovan	Novartis	Valsartan
Guaifenesin/ Phenylpropanolamine	Various	Guaifenesin/Phenylpropanolamine
Oxycontin	Purdue	Oxycodone
Oxycodone/APAP	Various	Oxycodone/APAP
Evista	Lilly	Raloxifene
Lotrel	Novartis	Amlodipine/Benazepril
Gemfibrozil	Various	Gemfibrozil
Propranolol	Various	Propranolol
Lotrisone	Key	Clotrimazole/Betamethasone
Ceftin	Glaxo Wellcome	Cefuroxime
Amaryl	Hoech Mar R	Glimepiride
Avandia	SK-Beecham	Rosiglitazone maleate
Procardia XL	Pfizer	Nifedipine
Zyprexa	Lilly	Olanzapine
Terazosin	Various	Terazosin
Butalbital/APAP/Caffiene	Various	Butalbital/APAP/Caffiene
Glipizide	Various	Glipizide
Promethazine (tabs)	Various	Promethazine
Triamcinolone (topical)	Various	Triamcinolone
Alesse	Wyeth-Ayerst	Levonorgestrel/Ethinyl Estradiol

Brand Name	Manufacturer	Generic Name
Captopril	Various	Captopril
Humulin 70/30	Lilly	Human Insulin 70/30
Acyclovir	Various	Acyclovir
Methylphenidate	Various	Methylphenidate
Lescol	Novartis	Fluvastatin
Hyzaar	Merck	Losartan/HCTZ
Minocycline	Various	Minocycline
Relafen	SK Beecham	Nabumetone
Combivent	Boehr Ingel	Ipratropium/Albuterol
Metoclopramide	Various	Metoclopramide
Zestoretic	Zeneca	Lisinopril/HCTZ
Levothroid	Forest	Levothyroxine
Promethazine/Codeine	Various	Promethazine/Codeine
Serzone	B-M Squibb	Nefazodone
Spironolactone	Various	Spironolactone
Ortho-Cyclen	Ortho Pharm	Norgestimate/Ethinyl Estradiol
Cimetidine	Various	Cimetidine
Necon 1/35	Watson	Ethinyl Estradiol/Norethindrone
Roxicet	Roxane	Oxycodone/APAP
Detrol	Pharmacia-Upjohn	Tolterodine
Macrobid	Procter & Gamble	Nitrofurantoin
Klor-Con	Upsher-Smith	Potassium Chloride
Imitrex	Glaxo Wellcome	Sumatriptan
Baycol	Bayer	Cerivastatin
Bactroban	SK Beecham	Mupirocin
Cardizem CD	Hoech Mar R	Diltiazem
Nortriptyline	Various	Nortriptyline
Flomax	Abbott	Tamsulosin
Avapro	B-M Squibb	Irbesartan
Actos	Takeda	Pioglitazone
Lo/Ovral	Wyeth-Ayerst	Norgestrel/Ethinyl Estradiol
Altace	Monarch	Ramipril
Albuterol (Liquid)	Various	Albuterol
Miacalcin	Novartis	Calcitonin Salmon
Claritin Reditabs	Schering	Loratadine

Brand Name	Manufacturer	Generic Name
Atrovent	Boehr Ingel	Ipratropium
Naproxen Sodium	Various	Naproxen Sodium
Plendil	Astra	Felodipine
Clindamycin	Various	Clindamycin
Valtrex	Glaxo Wellcome	Valacyclovir
Tamoxifen	Various	Tamoxifen
Phenobarbital	Various	Phenobarbital
BuSpar	B-M Squibb	Buspirone
Tiazac	Forest	Diltiazem
Proventil HFA	Key	Albuterol
Azmacort	RPR Pharm	Triamcinolone aerosol
Phenazopyridine	Various	Phenazopyridine
Remeron	Organon	Mirtazapine
Benzonatate	Various	Benzonatate
Nitroglycerin	Various	Nitroglycerin
Theophylline SR	Various	Theophylline
Vicoprofen	Knoll	Hydrocodone/Ibuprofen
Ery-Tab	Abbott	Erythromycin
Loestrin Fe 1/20	Parke Davis	Norethindrone/Ethinyl Estradiol
Elocon	Schering	Mometasone
Diovan HCT	Novartis	Valsartan/HCTZ
Hyoscyamine	Various	Hyoscyamine
Doxepin	Various	Doxepin
Digoxin	Various	Digoxin
Aciphex	Eisai	Rabeprazole
Tobradex	Alcon	Tobramycin/Dexamethasone
Diclofenac Sodium	Various	Diclofenac
Zyrtec Syrup	Pfizer	Cetirizine
Mircette	Organon	Desogestrel/Ethinyl Estradiol
Methocarbamol	Various	Methocarbamol

Source: RXList.com

For information that is useful but general and won't impact your daily work, you should maintain a reference file. You would keep this file at home and place general pharmacy-related articles in it after you have read them.

For example, if you read an article about ATM-style prescription dispensing machines in the newspaper, you would cut it out and file it for future reference. This is not an article that will help you every day at work, but you might want to reread it at a later date.

IN THE NEWS

In an effort to combat potentially deadly drug errors, the U.S. Health Secretary announced a proposal that would require supermarket-style bar codes on all hospital-administered prescription medications. The bar codes would include information on the medications' properties and expiration dates. In addition, patients would wear wristbands with bar codes that would include their ailments and any allergies. At the time this book went to press, the regulation was not yet in place but is expected to be in 2002.

Source: The Associated Press

FINAL THOUGHTS

As noted throughout this book, there is a growing need for pharmacy technicians, and that need is unlikely to diminish anytime soon. Technicians are increasingly well-respected, especially certified pharmacy technicians. As regulations and education requirements become stiffer and more states require certification, certified pharmacy technicians will become even more respected. With that status will come increased pay and increased responsibilities, as well. It will be your responsibility, as someone who has chosen this career, to ensure that you make a positive contribution to the pharmacy technician vocation. Look for new ways to improve your skills and gain more knowledge. Understand that you are an important member of the healthcare industry and that your work makes a substantial impact on the world around you. It's a big responsibility and a big honor.

THE INSIDE TRACK

Who: Lucy Angelo

What: CPhT

Where: Tinger Geriatric Center

                  Denver, Colorado

When I graduated from high school in 1996, I wasn't exactly sure what I wanted to with myself. I was working at a local CVS as a cashier, and one of my friends was a tech in the pharmacy, and she really loved her job. She sold me on getting into the field, and advised me on the best way to put myself into a good position for securing a job when I was ready. I attended a Technician Certificate program at my local community college and graduated with honors in 1998. Shortly after graduation, I took the exam and became certified. But graduation and certification didn't stop my education—in the following years I took Compounding training and Aseptic Technique training. I think growing as a professional and giving myself options is important.

I got my current job, working in a geriatric hospital, very shortly after I graduated. One of my training program instructors works at the hospital and "recruited" me for the position. At the time, they were hiring three techs, and two of us came from the same training program. I didn't get certified until I was already three months on the job, and because of that, I didn't realize a higher pay until almost a year after I became certified. After a year, though, I was bumped up more than I would have been if I were not certified. Besides the higher salary, I also feel like I get more respect from the pharmacists. I've also been involved in special projects that one of the pharmacists I work under set up for me. These have been projects for recertification (you have to be recertified every 2 years) and I wouldn't be involved in them if it wasn't for certification. The projects have been great learning experiences for me.

When I started out, I didn't realize that I was beginning a career in such an exciting and growing field. Since I have become a pharmacy technician, there have been many advances in the pharmaceutical world. Every time I open the newspaper, it seems there is another story about a new drug or a new regulation. It is exciting to think that I am part of that industry.

I've also made a lot of good friends through a regional technician group. We have official meetings once a month but I see many of the techs outside of the meetings. This has been good for me because I learn about new regulations and events from them. And, we share stories and complaints (everyone has them—no matter how much they love their jobs!). We've formed a sort of support group and we do help each other out. For example, some of us are certified, but others aren't. When someone is preparing to take the exam, they have many resources in the group to help them study.

On the job, I compound lotions, creams, and ointments, and I'm also involved in chemotherapy preparation. I order drugs and supplies and maintain the technician schedule. I also check daily cart fills—a duty that, as a CPhT, I can perform. Non-certified technicians are not allowed to check daily cart fills. As a CPhT, I would advise all prospective technicians to become certified. There is a shortage of good, qualified, reliable technicians. In my experience, I have seen a large difference in the quality of certified and non-certified technicians. Certified pharmacy technicians have the ability to work better with pharmacists because they are more confident and knowledgeable. The pharmacists tend to trust their abilities more, so they have them perform tasks that they might not give to non-certified techs.

Personally, I enjoy being a pharmacy technician. It is interesting work and I like the flexibility. Right now, I work about 30 hours a week, which I love. I recommend that anyone interested in becoming a pharmacy technician do some research into it, they might just find their ideal career for life, like me!

Professional Associations

IN ADDITION to contact information for national and state pharmacy associations, this appendix lists the affiliated organizations of the National Association of Boards of Pharmacy.

NATIONAL ASSOCIATIONS

Academy of Managed Care Pharmacy
100 North Pitt Street, Suite 400
Alexandria, VA 22314
www.amcp.org

American Association of Colleges of
  Pharmacy
1426 Prince Street
Alexandria, VA 22314
703-739-2330
Fax: 703-836-8982
http://207.188.222.124/

American College of Clinical Pharmacy
World Headquarters
3101 Broadway, Suite 650
Kansas City, MO 64111
816-531-2177
Fax: 816-531-4990
www.accp.com

American Institute of the History of
  Pharmacy
The University of Wisconsin
School of Pharmacy
777 Highland Avenue
Madison, WI 53705-2222
608-262-5378
www.pharmacy.wisc.edu/aihp/

American Association of Pharmacy
  Technicians
P.O. Box 1447
Greensboro, NC 27402
877-368-4771
Fax: 336-275-7222
www.pharmacytechnician.com

American Association of Health-System
  Pharmacists
7272 Wisconsin Avenue
Bethesda, MD 20814
301-657-3000
www.ashp.org

American Pharmaceutical Association
2215 Constitution Avenue NW
Washington, DC 20037-2985
202-628-4410
Fax: 202-783-2351
www.aphanet.org

Canadian Society for Pharmaceutical
　Sciences
3118 Dentistry/Pharmacy Centre
University of Alberta Campus
Edmonton, Alberta, Canada, T6G 2N8
780-492-0950
Fax: 780-492-0951
www.ualberta.ca/~csps/index.htm

Drug Information Association
501 Office Center Drive, Suite 450
Fort Washington, PA 19034-3211
215-628-2288
Fax: 215-641-1229
www.diahome.org

The International Academy of Compounding
　Pharmacists
P.O. Box 1365
Sugar Land, TX 77487
281-933-8400 or 800-927-4227
Fax: 281-495-0602
www.iacprx.org

Kappa Psi Pharmaceutical Fraternity
The Central Office
Southwestern Oklahoma State University
　School of Pharmacy
100 Campus Drive
Weatherford, OK 73096
580-774-7170
www.kappa-psi.org

National Association of Boards of Pharmacy
700 Busse Highway
Park Ridge, IL 60068
847-698-6227
Fax: 847-698-0124
www.nabp.net

National Community Pharmacists
　Association
205 Daingerfield Road
Alexandria, VA 22314
703-683-8200 or 800-544-7447
Fax: 703-683-3619
www.ncpanet.org

Pharmacy Technician Certification Board
2215 Constitution Avenue NW
Washington, DC 20037-2985
202-429-7576
Fax: 202-429-7596
www.pctb.org

Pharmacy Technician Educators Council
7060 South Brook Forest Drive
Evergreen, CO 80439
800-798-3247
www.rxptec.org

National Pharmacy Technician Association
P.O. Box 683148
Houston, TX 77268-3148
888-247-8700
Fax: 281-895-7320
www.pharmacytechnician.org

National Association of Chain Drug Stores

413 North Lee Street

P.O. Box 1417

Alexandria, VA 22313-1480

703-549-3001

Fax: 703-836-4869

www.nacds.org

STATE ASSOCIATIONS

Alabama Pharmacy Association

1211 Carmichael Way

Montgomery, AL 36106

334-271-4222; 800-529-7533

www.aparx.org

Alaska Pharmaceutical Association

P.O. Box 101185

Anchorage, AK 99510

907-563-8880

www.alaskapharmacy.org

Arizona Pharmacy Association

1845 East Southern Avenue

Tempe, AZ 85282

480-838-3385

Fax: 480-838-3557

www.azpharmacy.org

Arkansas Pharmacists Association

417 South Victory Street

Little Rock, AR 72201

501-372-5250

Fax: 501-372-0546

www.arpharmacists.org

California Pharmacists Association

1112 I Street, Suite 300

Sacramento, CA 95814

916-444-7811

Fax: 916-444-7929

www.calpharm.com

Florida Pharmacy Association

610 North Adams Street

Tallahassee, FL 32301

850-222-2400

Fax: 850-561-6758

www.pharmview.com

Georgia Pharmacy Association

50 Lenox Pointe, NE

Atlanta, GA 30324

404-231-5074

Fax: 404-237-8435

www.gpha.org

Illinois Council of Health-System
  Pharmacists
4430 Manchester Drive, Suite G-2
Rockford, IL 61109-1656
815-227-9292
Fax: 815-227-9294
www.ichpnet.org

Indiana Pharmacists Alliance
729 North Pennsylvania Street
Indianapolis, IN 46204
317-634-4968
Fax: 317-632-1219
www.indianapharmacists.org

Iowa Pharmacy Association
8515 Douglas Avenue, Suite 16
Des Moines, IA 50322
515-270-0713
Fax: 515-270-2979
www.iarx.org

Kansas Pharmacists Association
1020 SW Fairlawn Road
Topeka, KS 66604
785-228-2327
Fax: 785-228-9147
www.kansaspharmacy.org

Michigan Pharmacists Association
815 North Washington Avenue
Lansing, MI 48906-5198
517-484-1466
Fax: 517-484-5198
www.mipharm.com

Minnesota Pharmacists Association
1935 West County Road, B2 #450
Roseville, MN 55113
651-697-1771
Fax: 651-697-1776
www.mpha.org

Missouri Pharmacy Association
211 East Capitol
Jefferson City, MO 65101
www.morx.com

Nevada Pharmacists Association
3660 Baker Lane, #204
Reno, NV 89509
702-826-3981
Fax: 702-825-0785
www.wcmsnv.org

New Mexico Society of Health-System
  Pharmacists
P.O. Box 93550
Albuquerque, NM 87199-3550
505-856-0281
Fax: 505-856-0282
www.nmshp.org

Pharmacists Society of the State of
  New York
210 Washington Avenue Extension
Albany, NY 12203
800-632-8822 or 518-869-6595
Fax: 518-464-0618
www.pssny.org

North Carolina Association of Pharmacists
109 Church Street
Chapel Hill, NC 27516
919-967-2237
Fax: 919-968-9430
www.ncpharmacists.org

Ohio Pharmacists Association
6037 Frantz Road
Suite 106 Dublin, OH 43017
614-798-0037
Fax: 614-798-0978
www.ohiopharmacists.org
E-mail: info@ohiopharmacists.org

Oklahoma Society of Health-System
   Pharmacists
P.O. Box 18731
Oklahoma City, OK 73154
www.oshp.net

Pennsylvania Pharmacists Association
508 North Third Street
Harrisburg, PA 17101-1199
717-234-6151
www.papharmacists.com

Pharmacy Society of Wisconsin
701 Heartland Trail
Madison, WI 53717
608-827-9200
Fax: 608-827-9292
www.pswi.org

Rhode Island Pharmacists Association
Independent Square
500 Prospect Street
Pawtucket, RI 02860
401-725-4141
Fax: 401-725-9960
www.ripharm.com

South Dakota Pharmacists Association
P.O. Box 518
Pierre, SD 57501
605-224-2338
Fax: 605-224-1280
www.sdpha.org

Tennessee Pharmacists Association
226 Capitol Boulevard, Suite 810
Nashville, TN 37219-1893
615-256-3023
Fax: 615-255-3528
www.tnpharm.org

Texas Pharmacy Association
P.O. Box 14709
Austin, TX 78761-4709
800-505-5463 or 512-836-8350
www.txpharmacy.com

Utah Pharmaceutical Association
1850 South Columbia Lane
Orem, UT 84097
801-762-0452
Fax: 801-762-0454
www.upha.com

Virginia Pharmacists Association
5501 Patterson Avenue, Suite 200
Richmond, VA 23226
800-527-8742
Fax: 804-285-4227
http://pharmacy.su.edu

Wyoming Pharmacists Association
P.O. Box 2109
Glenrock, WY 82637
307-766-6988
Fax: 307-766-2953
www.wpha.net

Washington State Pharmacists Association
1501 Taylor Ave, SW
Renton, WA 98055-3139
425-228-7171; 425-277-3897
www.pharmcare.org

Washington State Pharmacists Association
1501 Taylor Ave, SW
Renton, WA 98055-3139
425-228-7171; 425-277-3897
www.pharmcare.org

BOARDS OF PHARMACY

Alabama State Board of Pharmacy
1 Perimeter Park South
Suite 425 South
Birmingham, AL 35243
205-967-0130
www.albop.com

Alaska Board of Pharmacy
P.O. Box 110806
Juneau, AK 99811-0806
907-465-2589
www.dced.state.ak.us/occ/ppha.htm

Arizona State Board of Pharmacy
4425 W. Olive Avenue, Suite 140
Glendale, AZ 85302
623-463-2727
www.pharmacy.state.az.us
E-mail: info@azsbp.com

Arkansas State Board of Pharmacy
101 East Capitol, Suite 218
Little Rock, AR 72201
501-682-0190
www.state.ar.us/asbp

California State Board of Pharmacy
400 R Street, Suite 4070
Sacramento, CA 95814
916-445-5014
www.pharmacy.ca.gov/

Colorado State Board of Pharmacy
1560 Broadway, Suite 1310
Denver, CO 80202
303-894-7750
www.dora.state.co.us/pharmacy

Connecticut Commission of Pharmacy
State Office Building
165 Capitol Avenue, Room 147
Hartford, CT 06106
860-713-6070
Fax 860-713-7242
www.ctdrugcontrol.com/rxcommision.htm

Delaware State Board of Pharmacy
P.O. Box 637
Dover, DE 19901
302-739-4798

District of Columbia Board of Pharmacy
825 North Capitol Street, N.E.
Room 2224
Washington, DC 20002
202-442-9200
Fax 202-442-9431

Florida Board of Pharmacy
4052 Bald Cypress Way, Bin #C04
Tallahassee, FL 32399-3254
850-245-4292
www9.myflorida.com/mqa/pharmacy/
    2001ph_home.html

Georgia State Board of Pharmacy
237 Coliseum Drive
Macon, GA 31217-3858
478-207-1686
www.sos.state.ga.us/ebd-pharmacy

Guam Board of Examiners for Pharmacy
P.O. Box 2816
Hagatna, GU 96932
671-475-0251

Hawaii State Board of Pharmacy
P.O. Box 3469
Honolulu, HI 96801
808-586-2694
www.state.hi.us/dcca/pvl/

Idaho Board of Pharmacy
P.O. Box 83720
Boise, ID 83720-0067
208-334-2356
www.state.id.us/bop

Illinois Department of Professional
    Regulation—State Board of Pharmacy
320 West Washington Street
Third Floor
Springfield, IL 62786
217-785-8159
www.dpr.state.il.us

Indiana Board of Pharmacy
402 W. Washington Street, Room 041
Indianapolis, IN 46204-2739
317-234-2067
www.in.gov/hpb/boards/isbp/

Iowa Board of Pharmacy Examiners
400 S.W. Eighth Street, Suite E
Des Moines, IA 50309-4688
515-281-5944
www.state.ia.us/ibpe

Kansas State Board of Pharmacy
Landon State Office Building
900 Jackson, Room 513
Topeka, KS 66612
785-296-4056
www.ink.org/public/pharmacy

Kentucky Board of Pharmacy
23 Millcreek Park
Frankfort, KY 40601-9230
502-573-1580
Fax: 502-573-1582
www.state.ky.us/boards/pharmacy

Louisiana Board of Pharmacy
5615 Corporate Boulevard, Suite 8E
Baton Rouge, LA 70808-2537
225-925-6496
www.labp.com

Maine Board of Pharmacy
35 State House Station
Augusta, ME 04333
207-624-8603 or Direct Line: 207-624-8620
Fax: 207-624-8637
Hearing Impaired: 207-624-8563
www.state.me.us/pfr/olr/

Maryland Board of Pharmacy
4201 Patterson Avenue
Baltimore, MD 21215-2299
410-764-4755
www.dhmh.state.md.us/pharmacyboard/
E-mail: md_pharmacy_board@yahoo.com

Massachusetts Board of Registration in
    Pharmacy
239 Causeway Street
Boston, MA 02113
617-727-9953
www.state.ma.us/reg/boards/ph

Michigan Board of Pharmacy
611 West Ottawa, First Floor
P.O. Box 30670,
Lansing, MI 48909-8170
517-373-9102
www.cis.state.mi.us

Minnesota Board of Pharmacy
David E. Holmstrom, Executive Director
2829 University Avenue SE, Suite 530
Minneapolis, MN 55414-3251
612-617-2201
www.phcybrd.state.mn.us
E-mail: pharmacy.board@state.mn.us

Mississippi State Board of Pharmacy
P.O. Box 24507
Jackson, MS 39225-4507
601-354-6750
www.mbp.state.ms.us

Missouri Board of Pharmacy
P.O. Box 625
Jefferson City, MO 65102
573-751-0091
www.ecodev.state.mo.us/pr/pharmacy

Montana Board of Pharmacy
P.O. Box 200513
111 North Jackson
Helena, MT 59620-0513
406-841-2356
Fax: 406-841-2343
www.com.state.mt.us/License/POL/
    pol_boards/pha_board/board_page.htm

Nebraska Board of Pharmacy
P.O. Box 94986
Lincoln, NE 68509
402-471-2115
www.hhs.state.ne.us

Nevada State Board of Pharmacy
555 Double Eagle Court, Suite 1100
Reno, NV 89511-8991
775-850-1440
www.state.nv.us/pharmacy

New Hampshire Board of Pharmacy
57 Regional Drive
Concord, NH 03301-8518
603-271-2350
www.state.nh.us/pharmacy
E-mail: nhpharmacy@nhsa.state.nh.us

New Jersey State Board of Pharmacy
P.O. Box 45013
Newark, NJ 07101
973-504-6450
www.state.nj.us/lps/ca/brief/pharm.htm

New Mexico Board of Pharmacy
1650 University Boulevard N.E.
Suite 400B
Albuquerque, NM 87102
505-841-9102
www.state.nm.us/pharmacy
E-mail: nmbop@nm-us.campuscwix.net.

New York Board of Pharmacy
89 Washington Avenue
Second Floor West
Albany, NY 12234-1000
518-474-3817 ext.130
Fax: 518-473-6995
www.nysed.gov/prof/pharm.htm
E-mail: pharmbd@mail.nysed.gov.

North Carolina Board of Pharmacy
P.O. Box 459
Carrboro, NC 27510-0459
919-942-4454
www.ncbop.org

North Dakota State Board of Pharmacy
P.O. Box 1354
Bismarck, ND 58502-1354
701-328-9535

Ohio State Board of Pharmacy
77 South High Street, Room 1702
Columbus, OH 43215-6126
614-466-4143
www.state.oh.us/pharmacy/

Oklahoma State Board of Pharmacy
4545 Lincoln Boulevard, Suite 112
Oklahoma City, OK 73105-3488
405-521-3815
www.state.ok.us/~pharmacy
E-mail: pharmacy@oklaosf.state.ok.us.

Oregon State Board of Pharmacy
800 N.E. Oregon Street, #9
State Office Building, Room 425
Portland, OR 97232
503-731-4032
www.pharmacy.state.or.us
E-mail: pharmacy.board@state.or.us.

Pennsylvania State Board of Pharmacy
124 Pine Street
P.O. Box 2649
Harrisburg, PA 17105-2649
717-783-7156
www.dos.state.pa.us/bpoa/phabd/
    mainpage.htm

Puerto Rico Board of Pharmacy
800 Avenida Robert T. Todd
Office #201, Stop 18
Santurce, PR 00908
787-725-8161

Rhode Island Board of Pharmacy
3 Capitol Hill, Room 205
Providence, RI 02908
401-222-2837

South Carolina Department of Labor,
    Licensing and Regulation—Board of
    Pharmacy
P.O. Box 11927
Columbia, SC 29211-1927
803-896-4700
www.llr.state.sc.us

South Dakota State Board of Pharmacy
4305 S. Louise Avenue, Suite 104
Sioux Falls, SD 57106
605-362-2737
Fax: 605-362-2738
www.state.sd.us/dcr/pharmacy

Tennessee Board of Pharmacy
Second Floor, Davy Crockett Tower
500 James Robertson Parkway
Nashville, TN 37243
615-741-2718
www.state.tn.us/commerce/pharmacy

Texas State Board of Pharmacy
333 Guadalupe, Tower 3, Suite 600, Box 21
Austin, TX 78701-3942
512-305-8000
www.tsbp.state.tx.us

Utah Board of Pharmacy
160 E. 300 South
P.O. Box 146741
Salt Lake City, UT 84114-6741
801-530-6767
www.commerce.state.ut.us/dopl/dopl1.htm
(through Division of Occupational and
    Professional Licensing)

Vermont Board of Pharmacy
26 Terrace Street, Drawer 09
Montpelier, VT 05609-1106
802-828-2875
www.vtprofessionals.org/pharmacists
E-mail: cpreston@sec.state.vt.us

Virgin Islands Board of Pharmacy
Roy L. Schneider Hospital
48 Sugar Estate
St. Thomas, VI 00802
340-774-0117

Virginia Board of Pharmacy
Elizabeth Scott Russell, Executive Director
6606 W. Broad Street, Suite 400
Richmond, VA 23230-1717
804-662-9911
www.dhp.state.va.us/pharmacy/default.htm

Washington State Board of Pharmacy
P.O. Box 47863
Olympia, WA 98504-7863
360-236-4825
www.doh.wa.gov/pharmacy/

West Virginia Board of Pharmacy
232 Capitol Street, Charleston, WV 25301
304-558-0558

Wisconsin Pharmacy Examining Board
1400 E. Washington
P.O. Box 8935,
Madison, WI 53708
608-266-2812
www.state.wi.us/agencies/drl

Wyoming State Board of Pharmacy
1720 S. Poplar Street, Suite 4
Casper, WY 82601
307-234-0294
http://pharmacyboard.state.wy.us

CANADIAN ASSOCIATIONS

Alberta Pharmaceutical Association
10130 112th Street, 7th Floor
Edmonton, Alberta
Canada T5K 2K4
780-990-0321

College of Pharmacists of British Columbia
200 1765 W. 8th Avenue
Vancouver, BC
Canada V6J 1V8
604-733-2440
www.collpharmbc.org

Manitoba Pharmaceutical Association
187 Saint Mary's Road
Winnipeg, Manitoba
Canada R2H 1J2
204-233-1411

New Brunswick Pharmaceutical Society
30 Gordon Street, Suite 101
Moncton, NB
Canada E1C 1L8
506-857-8957

Newfoundland Pharmaceutical Association
Apothecary Hall
488 Water Street
St. John's, Newfoundland
Canada A1E 1B3
709-753-5877

Nova Scotia Pharmaceutical Society
1526 Dresden Row
P.O. Box 3363 (South)
Halifax, NS
Canada B3J 3J1
902-422-8528

Ontario College of Pharmacists
483 Huron Street
Toronto, Ontario
Canada M5R 2R4
416-962-4861
www.ocpharma.com

Prince Edward Island Pharmacy Board
P.O. Box 89
Crapaud, PEI
Canada C0A 1J0
902-658-2780

Quebec Order of Pharmacists
266, rue Notre-Dame Ouest
Bureau 301
Montreal, Quebec
Canada H2Y 1T6
514-284-9588
www.opq.org
E-mail: ordrepharm@opq.org

Pharmacy Examining Board of Canada
123 Edward Street, Suite 603
Toronto, Ontario
Canada M5G 1E2
416-979-2431

National Association of Pharmacy
   Regulatory Authorities
402-222 Somerset Street, West
Ottawa, Ontario
Canada K2P 2G3
613-569-9658
www.napra.org

Additional Resources

FOR ADDITIONAL information on the topics discussed in this book, as well as helpful job-hunting information, refer to the following publications and online resources listed below. At the time of this book's publication, all the websites listed below were current. Unfortunately, due to the ever-changing face of the Web, we cannot guarantee every site will be in existence.

PUBLICATIONS

General Information

APhA's Complete Review for the Pharmacy Technician. L. Michael Posey. (Washington, DC: American Pharmaceutical Association, 2001).

APhA's Complete Math Review for the Pharmacy Technician. William A. Hopkins Jr. (Washington, DC: American Pharmaceutical Association, 2001).

Pharmacy Technician. Robert P. Shrewsbury. (Englewood, CO: Morton, 1999).

Pharmacy Technician Workbook & Certification. Joseph Medina. (Albany, NY: Delmar, 1999).

The Pharmacy Technician. Marvin M. Stoogenke. (Upper Saddle River, NJ: Prentice Hall, 1997).

On the Job

101 Ways to Improve Your Pharmacy Worklife. Mark R. Jacobs. (Washington, DC: American Pharmaceutical Association, 2001).

Essential Spanish for Pharmacists. Glenn R. Kisch. (Washington, DC: American Pharmaceutical Association, 1999).

The Pharmacy Technician Companion: Your Road Map to Technician and Careers. Linda R. Harteker, Jeffery J. Ball, and Julian I. Graubart. American Pharmaceutical Association (Washington, DC), 1998.

The Pharmacy Technician's Pocket Drug Reference. Joyce A. Generali. American Pharmaceutical Association (Washington, DC), 2001.

Saunders Pharmaceutical Word Book, 2001. Ellen Drake and Randy Drake. (Philadelphia, PA: WB Saunders 2001).

Finding the Right College & Paying for It

Best 331 Colleges: 2001 Edition. (New York: Princeton Review, 2001).

The College Board College Cost & Financial Aid Handbook 2001. (New York: College Entrance Examination Board, 2000).

The College Board Index of Majors and Graduate Degrees 2001. (New York: College Entrance Examination Board, 2000).

Kaplan Guide to the Best Colleges in the U.S. 2001. (New York: Kaplan Publishing, 2000).

Occupational Outlook Handbook. (Washington, DC: U.S. Department of Labor, 2001).

Peterson's Guide to Two-Year Colleges 1998: The Only Guide to More than 1,500 Community and Junior Colleges. (Lawrenceville, NJ: Peterson's Guides, 1998).

The Scholarship Book 2001: The Complete Guide to Private-Sector Scholarships, Fellowships, Grants, and Loans for the Undergraduate. Daniel J. Cassidy. (Upper Saddle River, NJ: Prentice Hall, 2000).

ONLINE JOB HUNTING

The Web is an extremely powerful job search tool that can not only help you find exciting job opportunities, but also research companies, network with other people in your field, and obtain valuable career-related advice.

Using any Internet search engine or portal, you can enter keywords such as: "resume," "pharmacy technicians jobs," "pharmacy technicians career," "pharmacy technicians job listings," or "help wanted" to find thousands of websites of interest to you. The following is a listing of just some of the online resources available to you.

Career Related Websites

▶ Best Jobs USA—www.bestjobsusa.com
▶ 1st Impressions Career Site—www.1st-imp.com
▶ About.com—www.jobsearch.about.com/jobs/jobsearch/msubrespost.htm
▶ Advanced Career Systems—www.resumesystems.com
▶ America's Employers—www.americasemployers.com
▶ Career & Resume Management for the 21st Century—www.crm21.com
▶ Career Builder—www.careerbuilder.com
▶ Career Center—www.jobweb.org
▶ Career Creations—www.careercreations.com
▶ Career.com—www.career.com
▶ CareerMosaic—www.careermosaic.com
▶ CareerNet—www.careers.org
▶ CareerWeb—www.cweb.com
▶ College Central Network—www.employercentral.com
▶ First Job: The Web Site—www.firstjob.com
▶ Gary Will's Work Search—www.garywill.com/worksearch
▶ JobBank USA—www.jobbankusa.com
▶ JobSource—www.jobsource.com
▶ JobStar—www.jobsmart.org/tools/resume
▶ JobTrack—www.jobtrack.com
▶ Kaplan Online Career Center—www.kaplan.com
▶ My Job Coach—www.myjobcoach.com
▶ National Business Employment Weekly Online—www.nbew.com
▶ Salary.com—www.salary.com
▶ The Boston Herald's Job Find—www.jobfind.com

▶ The Employment Guide's Career Web—www.cweb.com/jobs/resume.html

▶ The Monster Board —www.monster.com

▶ The Wall Street Journal Careers—www.careers.wsj.com

▶ Vault.com—www.vaultreports.com/jobBoard/SearchJobs.cfm

▶ Yahoo Careers—www.careers.yahoo.com

Most of these sites list only jobs in the healthcare professions; however a few of them are more comprehensive. Use the search term "pharmacy technician" to come up with a list of only those job openings that will be of interest to you.

Pharmaceutical Employment Sites

▶ America's Healthcare Source—www.healthcaresource.com

▶ Cardinal Health Staffing Network—www.pharmacistsprn.com

▶ Health Care Job Store—www.healthcarejobstore.com

▶ Healthcare Match—www.healthcarematch.com

▶ Healthcarejobs.net—www.healthcarejobs.net

▶ Hospital Network—www.hospitalnetwork.com

▶ HospitalHub.com—www.hospitalhub.com

▶ Med Explorer—www.medexplorer.com

▶ Med Health Jobs.com—www.medhealthjobs.com

▶ Medbulletin.com—www.medbulletin.com

▶ Medhunters.com—www.medhunters.com

▶ Medical Matrix—www.medicalmatrix.com

▶ Monster.com Healthcare—www.medsearch.com

▶ Pharmaceutical Online—www.pharmaceuticalonline.com

▶ Pharmacy Week—www.pharmacyweek.com

▶ Pharmahorizons.com—www.pharmahorizons.com

▶ RX Career Center.com—www.rxcareercenter.com

▶ Sierra Recruitment.com—www.healthcarecareers.com

Websites for Pharmacy Technician Education Programs

HERE YOU will find a list of popular and relevant websites from which to begin your search for a pharmacy technician education program. Finding the right school and program is important, so be sure to make time for a serious investigation of each of site and their corresponding links to different programs.

In addition to the links found here, check with your state Board of Pharmacy, which usually will have information on programs. Most counties and cities have local associations as well, or check with a local pharmacy organization that is affiliated with one of the national associations. For a complete listing of national organizations, state associations, and Boards of Pharmacy, see Appendix A.

www.aacp.org (American Association of Colleges of Pharmacy)
American Association of Colleges of Pharmacy, although not specifically recommending any particular school, provides a comprehensive Pharmacy Schools Directory. Organized by state, it lists names, addresses, and phone numbers of schools, with website and/or e-mail hotlinks to some. To find the list, select the "Pharmacy Schools" link on the left ear of their homepage.

www.petersons.com
Peterson's College Quest program provides the opportunity for a personalized search through a database of thousands of colleges and universities. You can select a field of study, such as "Pharmacy", then narrow the search by other criteria such as location and cost. A list of schools that meet your criteria will be displayed, providing detailed information about each school, including links to websites.

www.collegeview.com

This is another self-selecting search site, including over 3,000 colleges and universities. It includes information on each school and links to school websites.

www.embark.com

You can select your own criteria to search on this site which includes a business school section as well as colleges and universities. Detailed information and website links for each school are included.

www.collegecenter.com

This site provides advice regarding the selecting of appropriate colleges and universities and free information about the admissions process, but it charges fees for specific guidance services.

www.rwm.org/rwm

A database of private post-secondary vocational schools. The viewer selects a state, then a field of training. The displayed list shows school name, address, and telephone number, and a link to the school's website.

www.collegescolleges.com
www.ecola.com/college
www.megamallandmall.com/college.html
www.ulinks.com

Each of these sites provide names-only lists of colleges and universities arranged by state, with a hotlink to each school's website.

www.universities.com

This site offers lists of over 7,500 colleges and universities, arranged alphabetically or by state. Includes detailed information on schools and links to their websites.

Sample Free Application for Federal Student Aid (FAFSA)

ON THE following pages you will find a sample FAFSA. Use this form to familiarize yourself with the form so that when you apply for federal, and state student grants, work-study, and loans you will know what information you need to have ready. When this book went to press, this was the most current form, and although the form remains mostly the same from year to year, you should check the FAFSA website (www.fafsa.ed.gov) for the most current information.

2001-2002

The FAFSA

July 1, 2001 — June 30, 2002
Free Application for Federal Student Aid

OMB # 1845-0001

Use this form to apply for federal and state* student grants, work-study, and loans.

Apply over the Internet with 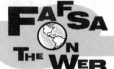 **www.fafsa.ed.gov**

 If you are filing a **2000 income tax return,** we recommend that you complete it before filling out this form. However, you do not need to file your income tax return with the IRS before you submit this form.

If you or your family has **unusual circumstances** (such as loss of employment) that might affect your need for student financial aid, submit this form, and then consult with the financial aid office at the college you plan to attend.

You may also use this form to apply for **aid from other sources, such as your state or college.** The deadlines for states (see table to right) or colleges may be as early as January 2001 and may differ. You may be required to complete additional forms. Check with your high school guidance counselor or a financial aid administrator at your college about state and college sources of student aid.

 Your answers on this form will be read electronically. Therefore:

- use black ink and fill in ovals completely:
- print clearly in CAPITAL letters and skip a box between words:
- report dollar amounts (such as $12,356.41) like this:

Yes ● No ⊗ ⊘

| I | 5 | | E | L | M | | S | T |

$ | 1 | 2 | , | 3 | 5 | 6 | no cents

Green is for students and purple is for parents.

If you have questions about this application, or for more information on eligibility requirements and the U.S. Department of Education's student aid programs, look on the Internet at **www.ed.gov/studentaid** You can also call 1-800-4FED-AID (1-800-433-3243) seven days a week from 8:00 a.m. through midnight (Eastern time). TTY users may call 1-800-730-8913.

 After you complete this application, make a copy of it for your records. Then **send the original of pages 3 through 6** in the attached envelope or send it to: Federal Student Aid Programs, P.O. Box 4008, Mt. Vernon, IL 62864-8608.

You should submit your application as early as possible, but no earlier than January 1, 2001. We must receive your application **no later than July 1, 2002.** Your school must have your correct, complete information by your last day of enrollment in the 2001-2002 school year.

You should hear from us within four weeks. If you do not, please call 1-800-433-3243 or check on-line at www.fafsa.ed.gov

 Now go to page 3 and begin filling out this form.
Refer to the notes as needed.

STATE AID DEADLINES

AR April 1, 2001 *(date received)*
AZ June 30, 2002 *(date received)*
*^ CA March 2, 2001 *(date postmarked)*
* DC June 24, 2001 *(date received by state)*
DE April 15, 2001 *(date received)*
FL May 15, 2001 *(date processed)*
HI March 1, 2001
^ IA July 1, 2001 *(date received)*
IL First-time applicants – September 30, 2001
    Continuing applicants – July 15, 2001
    (date received)
^ IN For priority consideration – March 1, 2001
    (date postmarked)
* KS For priority consideration – April 1, 2001
    (date received)
KY For priority consideration – March 15, 2001
    (date received)
^ LA For priority consideration – April 15, 2001
    Final deadline – July 1, 2001
    (date received)
^ MA For priority consideration – May 1, 2001
    (date received)
MD March 1, 2001 *(date postmarked)*
ME May 1, 2001 *(date received)*
MI High school seniors – February 21, 2001
    College students – March 21, 2001
    (date received)
MN June 30, 2002 *(date received)*
MO April 1, 2001 *(date received)*
MT For priority consideration – March 1, 2001
    (date postmarked)
NC March 15, 2001 *(date received)*
ND April 15, 2001 *(date processed)*
NH May 1, 2001 *(date received)*
^ NJ June 1, 2001 if you received a
    Tuition Aid Grant in 2000-2001
    All other applicants
    – October 1, 2001, for fall and spring terms
    – March 1, 2002, for spring term only
    (date received)
*^ NY May 1, 2002 *(date postmarked)*
OH October 1, 2001 *(date received)*
OK For priority consideration – April 30, 2001
    Final deadline – June 30, 2001
    (date received)
OR May 1, 2002 *(date received)*
* PA All 2000-2001 State Grant recipients and all
    non-2000-2001 State Grant recipients in
    degree programs – May 1, 2001
    All other applicants – August 1, 2001
    (date received)
PR May 2, 2002 *(date application signed)*
RI March 1, 2001 *(date received)*
SC June 30, 2001 *(date received)*
TN May 1, 2001 *(date processed)*
*^ WV March 1, 2001 *(date received)*

Check with your financial aid administrator for these states: AK, AL, *AS, *CT, CO, *FM, GA, *GU, ID, *MH, *MP, MS, *NE, *NM, *NV, *PW, *SD, *TX, UT, *VA, *VI, *VT, WA, WI, and *WY.

^ *Applicants encouraged to obtain proof of mailing.*
* *Additional form may be required*

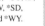

Notes for questions 13–14 (page 3)

If you are an eligible noncitizen, write in your eight or nine digit Alien Registration Number. Generally, you are an eligible noncitizen if you are: (1) a U.S. permanent resident and you have an Alien Registration Receipt Card (I-551); (2) a conditional permanent resident (I-551C); or (3) an other eligible noncitizen with an Arrival-Departure Record (I-94) from the U.S. Immigration and Naturalization Service showing any one of the following designations: "Refugee," "Asylum Granted," "Indefinite Parole," "Humanitarian Parole," or "Cuban-Haitian Entrant." If you are in the U.S. on only an F1 or F2 student visa, or only a J1 or J2 exchange visitor visa, or a G series visa (pertaining to international organizations), you must fill in oval c. If you are neither a citizen nor eligible noncitizen, you are not eligible for federal student aid. However, you may be eligible for state or college aid.

Notes for questions 17–21 (page 3)

For undergraduates, full time generally means taking at least 12 credit hours in a term or 24 clock hours per week. 3/4 time generally means taking at least 9 credit hours in a term or 18 clock hours per week. Half time generally means taking at least 6 credit hours in a term or 12 clock hours per week. Provide this information about the college you plan to attend.

Notes for question 29 (page 3) — Enter the correct number in the box in question 29.

Enter **1** for 1st bachelor's degree
Enter **2** for 2nd bachelor's degree
Enter **3** for associate degree (occupational or technical program)
Enter **4** for associate degree (general education or transfer program)
Enter **5** for certificate or diploma for completing an occupational, technical, or educational program of less than two years

Enter **6** for certificate or diploma for completing an occupational, technical, or educational program of at least two years
Enter **7** for teaching credential program (nondegree program)
Enter **8** for graduate or professional degree
Enter **9** for other/undecided

Notes for question 30 (page 3) — Enter the correct number in the box in question 30.

Enter **0** for 1st year undergraduate/never attended college
Enter **1** for 1st year undergraduate/attended college before
Enter **2** for 2nd year undergraduate/sophomore
Enter **3** for 3rd year undergraduate/junior

Enter **4** for 4th year undergraduate/senior
Enter **5** for 5th year/other undergraduate
Enter **6** for 1st year graduate/professional
Enter **7** for continuing graduate/professional or beyond

Notes for questions 37 c. and d. (page 4) and 71 c. and d. (page 5)

If you filed or will file a foreign tax return, or a tax return with Puerto Rico, Guam, American Samoa, the Virgin Islands, the Marshall Islands, the Federated States of Micronesia, or Palau, use the information from that return to fill out this form. If you filed a foreign return, convert all figures to U.S. dollars, using the exchange rate that is in effect today.

Notes for questions 38 (page 4) and 72 (page 5)

In general, a person is eligible to file a 1040A or 1040EZ if he or she makes less than $50,000, does not itemize deductions, does not receive income from his or her own business or farm, and does not receive alimony. A person is not eligible if he or she itemizes deductions, receives self-employment income or alimony, or is required to file Schedule D for capital gains.

Notes for questions 41 (page 4) and 75 (page 5) — only for people who filed a 1040EZ or Telefile

On the 1040EZ, if a person answered "Yes" on line 5, use EZ worksheet line F to determine the number of exemptions ($2,800 equals one exemption). If a person answered "No" on line 5, enter 01 if he or she is single, or 02 if he or she is married.

On the Telefile, use line J to determine the number of exemptions ($2,800 equals one exemption).

Notes for questions 47–48 (page 4) and 81–82 (page 5)

Net worth means current value minus debt. If net worth is one million or more, enter $999,999. If net worth is negative, enter 0.

Investments include real estate (do not include the home you live in), trust funds, money market funds, mutual funds, certificates of deposit, stocks, stock options, bonds, other securities, education IRAs, installment and land sale contracts (including mortgages held), commodities, etc. Investment value includes the market value of these investments as of today. Investment debt means only those debts that are related to the investments.

Investments do not include the home you live in, cash, savings, checking accounts, the value of life insurance and retirement plans (pension funds, annuities, noneducation IRAs, Keogh plans, etc.), or the value of prepaid tuition plans.

Business and/or investment farm value includes the market value of land, buildings, machinery, equipment, inventory, etc. Business and/or investment farm debt means only those debts for which the business or investment farm was used as collateral.

Notes for question 58 (page 4)

Answer **"No"** (you are not a veteran) if you (1) have never engaged in active duty in the U.S. Armed Forces, (2) are currently an ROTC student or a cadet or midshipman at a service academy, or (3) are a National Guard or Reserves enlistee activated only for training. Also answer "No" if you are currently serving in the U.S. Armed Forces and will continue to serve through June 30, 2002.

Answer **"Yes"** (you are a veteran) if you (1) have engaged in active duty in the U.S. Armed Forces (Army, Navy, Air Force, Marines, or Coast Guard) or as a member of the National Guard or Reserves who was called to active duty for purposes other than training, or were a cadet or midshipman at one of the service academies, **and** (2) were released under a condition other than dishonorable. Also answer "Yes" if you are not a veteran now but will be one by June 30, 2002.

Step One: For questions 1-34, leave blank any questions that do not apply to you (the student).

1-3. Your full name (as it appears on your Social Security Card)

| 1. LAST NAME | FOR INFORMATION ONLY | 2. FIRST NAME | DO NOT SUBMIT | 3. MIDDLE INITIAL |

4-7. Your permanent mailing address

4. NUMBER AND STREET (INCLUDE APT. NUMBER)

5. CITY (AND COUNTRY IF NOT U.S.)   6. STATE   7. ZIP CODE

8. Your Social Security Number
X X X – X X – X X X X

9. Your date of birth
/ / 1 9

10. Your permanent telephone number
( ) –

11-12. Your driver's license number and state (if any)

11. LICENSE NUMBER   12. STATE

13. Are you a U.S. citizen? Pick one. **See Page 2.**
- **a.** Yes, I am a U.S. citizen. .... ○ 1
- **b.** No, but I am an eligible noncitizen. **Fill in question 14.** ...... ○ 2
- **c.** No, I am not a citizen or eligible noncitizen. .... ○ 3

14. ALIEN REGISTRATION NUMBER
A

15. What is your marital status as of today?
- I am single, divorced, or widowed. ○ 1
- I am married/remarried. ○ 2
- I am separated. ○ 3

16. Month and year you were married, separated, divorced, or widowed
MONTH / YEAR

For each question (17 - 21), please mark whether you will be full time, 3/4 time, half time, less than half time, or not attending. **See page 2.**

17. Summer 2001 — Full time/Not sure ○ 1   3/4 time ○ 2   Half time ○ 3   Less than half time ○ 4   Not attending ○ 5
18. Fall 2001 — Full time/Not sure ○ 1   3/4 time ○ 2   Half time ○ 3   Less than half time ○ 4   Not attending ○ 5
19. Winter 2001-2002 — Full time/Not sure ○ 1   3/4 time ○ 2   Half time ○ 3   Less than half time ○ 4   Not attending ○ 5
20. Spring 2002 — Full time/Not sure ○ 1   3/4 time ○ 2   Half time ○ 3   Less than half time ○ 4   Not attending ○ 5
21. Summer 2002 — Full time/Not sure ○ 1   3/4 time ○ 2   Half time ○ 3   Less than half time ○ 4   Not attending ○ 5

22. Highest school your father completed — Middle school/Jr. High ○ 1   High school ○ 2   College or beyond ○ 3   Other/unknown ○ 4
23. Highest school your mother completed — Middle school/Jr. High ○ 1   High school ○ 2   College or beyond ○ 3   Other/unknown ○ 4

24. What is your state of legal residence? STATE

25. Did you become a legal resident of this state before January 1, 1996?   Yes ○ 1   No ○ 2

26. If the answer to question 25 is **"No,"** give month and year you became a legal resident.
MONTH / YEAR

27. Are you male? (Most male students must register with Selective Service to get federal aid.)   Yes ○ 1   No ○ 2
28. If you are male (age 18-25) and not registered, do you want Selective Service to register you?   Yes ○ 1   No ○ 2

29. What degree or certificate will you be working on during 2001-2002? **See page 2** and enter the correct number in the box.

30. What will be your grade level when you begin the 2001-2002 school year? **See page 2** and enter the correct number in the box.

31. Will you have a high school diploma or GED before you enroll?   Yes ○ 1   No ○ 2
32. Will you have your first bachelor's degree before July 1, 2001?   Yes ○ 1   No ○ 2
33. In addition to grants, are you interested in student loans (which you must pay back)?   Yes ○ 1   No ○ 2
34. In addition to grants, are you interested in "work-study" (which you earn through work)?   Yes ○ 1   No ○ 2

35. Do not leave this question blank. Have you ever been convicted of possessing or selling illegal drugs? If you have, answer "Yes," complete and submit this application, and we will send you a worksheet in the mail for you to determine if your conviction affects your eligibility for aid.
No ○ 1   Yes ○ 3

DO NOT LEAVE QUESTION 35 BLANK

Step Two: For questions 36-49, report your (the student's) income and assets. If you are married, report your spouse's income and assets, even if you were not married in 2000. Ignore references to "spouse" if you are currently single, separated, divorced, or widowed.

36. For 2000, have you (the student) completed your IRS income tax return or another tax return listed in **question 37**?

    a. I have already completed my return. ◯ ₁   **b.** I will file, but I have not yet ◯ ₂   **c.** I'm not going to file. **(Skip to question 42.)** ◯ ₃
                                                 completed my return.

37. What income tax return did you file or will you file for 2000?

    a. IRS 1040 .... ◯ ₁   **d.** A tax return for Puerto Rico, Guam, American Samoa, the Virgin Islands, the
    b. IRS 1040A, 1040EZ, 1040Telefile ...... ◯ ₂   Marshall Islands, the Federated States of Micronesia, or Palau. **See Page 2.** ...... ◯ ₄
    c. A foreign tax return. **See Page 2.** ...... ◯ ₃

38. If you have filed or will file a 1040, were you eligible to file a 1040A or 1040EZ? **See page 2.**   **Yes** ◯ ₁   **No** ◯ ₂   Don't Know ◯ ₃

For questions 39-51, if the answer is zero or the question does not apply to you, enter 0.

39. What was your (and spouse's) adjusted gross income for 2000? Adjusted gross income is on IRS Form 1040–line 33; 1040A–line 19; 1040EZ–line 4; or Telefile–line I. $ ⬚⬚⬚ , ⬚⬚⬚

40. Enter the total amount of your (and spouse's) income tax for 2000. Income tax amount is on IRS Form 1040–line 51; 1040A–line 33; 1040EZ–line 10; or Telefile–line K. $ ⬚⬚⬚ , ⬚⬚⬚

41. Enter your (and spouse's) exemptions for 2000. Exemptions are on IRS Form 1040–line 6d or on Form 1040A–line 6d. For Form 1040EZ or Telefile, **see page 2.**   ⬚⬚

42-43. How much did you (and spouse) earn from working in 2000? Answer this question whether or not you filed a tax return. This information may be on your W-2 forms, or on IRS Form 1040–lines 7 + 12 + 18; 1040A–line 7; or 1040EZ–line 1. Telefilers should use their W-2's.   **You (42)** $ ⬚⬚⬚ , ⬚⬚⬚

    Your Spouse (43) $ ⬚⬚⬚ , ⬚⬚⬚

Student (and Spouse) Worksheets (44-46)

44-46. Go to Page 8 and complete the columns on the left of Worksheets A, B, and C. Enter the student (and spouse) totals in questions 44, 45, and 46, respectively. Even though you may have few of the Worksheet items, check each line carefully.

    Worksheet A (44) $ ⬚⬚⬚ , ⬚⬚⬚

    Worksheet B (45) $ ⬚⬚⬚ , ⬚⬚⬚

    Worksheet C (46) $ ⬚⬚⬚ , ⬚⬚⬚

47. As of today, what is the net worth of your (and spouse's) current **investments**? **See page 2.** $ ⬚⬚⬚ , ⬚⬚⬚

48. As of today, what is the net worth of your (and spouse's) current **businesses and/or investment farms**? **See page 2.** Do not include a farm that you live on and operate. $ ⬚⬚⬚ , ⬚⬚⬚

49. As of today, what is your (and spouse's) total current balance of cash, savings, and checking accounts? $ ⬚⬚⬚ , ⬚⬚⬚

50-51. If you receive veterans education benefits, for **how many months** from July 1, 2001 through June 30, 2002 will you receive these benefits, and **what amount** will you receive per month? Do not include your spouse's veterans education benefits.   **Months (50)** ⬚⬚

    Amount (51) $ ⬚⬚⬚

Step Three: Answer all seven questions in this step.

52. Were you born before January 1, 1978? .... **Yes** ◯ ₁   **No** ◯ ₂

53. Will you be working on a master's or doctorate program (such as an MA, MBA, MD, JD, or Ph.D., etc.) during the school year 2001-2002? .... **Yes** ◯ ₁   **No** ◯ ₂

54. As of today, are you married? (Answer "Yes" if you are separated but not divorced.) .... **Yes** ◯ ₁   **No** ◯ ₂

55. Do you have children who receive more than half of their support from you? .... **Yes** ◯ ₁   **No** ◯ ₂

56. Do you have dependents (other than your children or spouse) who live with you and who receive more than half of their support from you, now and through June 30, 2002? .... **Yes** ◯ ₁   **No** ◯ ₂

57. Are you an orphan or ward of the court or were you a ward of the court until age 18? .... **Yes** ◯ ₁   **No** ◯ ₂

58. Are you a veteran of the U.S. Armed Forces? **See page 2.** .... **Yes** ◯ ₁   **No** ◯ ₂

If you (the student) answer "No" to every question in Step Three, go to Step Four.

If you answer "Yes" to any question in Step Three, skip Step Four and go to Step Five.

(If you are a graduate health profession student, your school may require you to complete Step Four even if you answered "Yes" in Step Three.)

Step Four: Complete this step if you (the student) answered "No" to all questions in Step Three.

59. **Go to page 7 to determine who is considered a parent for this step.** What is your parents' marital status as of today?

(Pick one.) Married/Remarried ○ ₁   Single ○ ₂   Divorced/Separated ○ ₃   Widowed ○

60-63. What are your parents' Social Security Numbers and last names?
If your parent does not have a Social Security Number, enter 000-00-0000

60. FATHER'S/STEPFATHER'S SOCIAL SECURITY NUMBER X X X – X X – X X X X

61. FATHER'S/STEPFATHER'S LAST NAME F O R I N F O R M A T I O N O N L Y

62. MOTHER'S/STEPMOTHER'S SOCIAL SECURITY NUMBER X X X – X X – X X X X

63. MOTHER'S/STEPMOTHER'S LAST NAME D O N O T S U B M I T

64. **Go to page 7** to determine how many people are in your parents' household.

65. **Go to page 7** to determine how many in question 64 **(exclude your parents)** will be college students between July 1, 2001 and June 30, 2002.

66. What is your parents' state of legal residence?   STATE

67. Did your parents become legal residents of the state in question 66 before January 1, 1996?   Yes ○ ₁   No ○

68. If the answer to question 67 is "No," give the month and year legal residency began for the parent who has lived in the state the longest.   MONTH / YEAR

69. What is the age of your older parent?

70. For 2000, have your parents completed their IRS income tax return or another tax return listed in **question 71**?

   a. My parents have already completed their return. ○ ₁   **b.** My parents will file, but they have not yet completed their return. ○ ₂   **c.** My parents are not going to file. **(Skip to question 76.)** ○

71. What income tax return did your parents file or will they file for 2000?

   a. IRS 1040 .... ○ ₁   **d.** A tax return for Puerto Rico, Guam, American Samoa, the Virgin Islands, the Marshall Islands, the Federated States of Micronesia, or Palau. **See Page 2.** .... ○
   b. IRS 1040A, 1040EZ, 1040Telefile ..... ○ ₂
   c. A foreign tax return. **See Page 2.** ...... ○ ₃

72. If your parents have filed or will file a 1040, were they eligible to file a 1040A or 1040EZ? **See page 2.**   Yes ○ ₁   No ○ ₂   Don't Know ○ ₃

For questions 73 - 83, if the answer is zero or the question does not apply, enter 0.

73. What was your parents' adjusted gross income for 2000? Adjusted gross income is on IRS Form 1040–line 33; 1040A–line 19; 1040EZ–line 4; or Telefile–line I. $

74. Enter the total amount of your parents' income tax for 2000. Income tax amount is on IRS Form 1040–line 51; 1040A–line 33; 1040EZ–line 10; or Telefile–line K. $

75. Enter your parents' exemptions for 2000. Exemptions are on IRS Form 1040–line 6d or on Form 1040A–line 6d. For Form 1040EZ or Telefile, **see page 2.**

76-77. How much did your parents earn from working in 2000? Answer this question whether or not your parents filed a tax return. This information may be on their W-2 forms, or on IRS Form 1040–lines 7 + 12 + 18; 1040A–line 7; or 1040EZ–line 1. Telefilers should use their W-2's.

   Father/ Stepfather (76) $
   Mother/ Stepmother (77) $

Parent Worksheets (78-80)

78-80. Go to Page 8 and complete the columns on the right of Worksheets A, B, and C. Enter the parent totals in questions 78, 79, and 80, respectively. Even though your parents may have few of the Worksheet items, check each line carefully.

   Worksheet A (78) $
   Worksheet B (79) $
   Worksheet C (80) $

81. As of today, what is the net worth of your parents' current **investments**? **See page 2.** $

82. As of today, what is the net worth of your parents' current **businesses and/or investment farms**? **See page 2.** Do not include a farm that your parents live on and operate. $

83. As of today, what is your parents' total current balance of cash, savings, and checking accounts? $

Now go to Step Six.

Step Five: Complete this step only if you (the student) answered "Yes" to any question in Step Three.

84. **Go to page 7** to determine how many people are in your (and your spouse's) household. ☐☐

85. **Go to page 7** to determine how many in question 84 will be college students between July 1, 2001 and June 30, 2002. ☐

Step Six: Please tell us which schools should receive your information.

For each school (up to six), please provide the federal school code and your housing plans. Look for the federal school codes on the Internet at **www.fafsa.ed.gov**, at your college financial aid office, at your public library, or by asking your high school guidance counselor. If you cannot get the federal school code, write in the complete name, address, city, and state of the college.

86. 1ST FEDERAL SCHOOL CODE ☐☐☐☐☐☐ OR — NAME OF COLLEGE — ADDRESS AND CITY — STATE ☐☐
HOUSING PLANS
87. on campus ○ 1 / off campus ○ 2 / with parent ○ 3

88. 2ND FEDERAL SCHOOL CODE ☐☐☐☐☐☐ OR — NAME OF COLLEGE — ADDRESS AND CITY — STATE ☐☐
89. on campus ○ 1 / off campus ○ 2 / with parent ○ 3

90. 3RD FEDERAL SCHOOL CODE ☐☐☐☐☐☐ OR — NAME OF COLLEGE — ADDRESS AND CITY — STATE ☐☐
91. on campus ○ 1 / off campus ○ 2 / with parent ○ 3

92. 4TH FEDERAL SCHOOL CODE ☐☐☐☐☐☐ OR — NAME OF COLLEGE — ADDRESS AND CITY — STATE ☐☐
93. on campus ○ 1 / off campus ○ 2 / with parent ○ 3

94. 5TH FEDERAL SCHOOL CODE ☐☐☐☐☐☐ OR — NAME OF COLLEGE — ADDRESS AND CITY — STATE ☐☐
95. on campus ○ 1 / off campus ○ 2 / with parent ○ 3

96. 6TH FEDERAL SCHOOL CODE ☐☐☐☐☐☐ OR — NAME OF COLLEGE — ADDRESS AND CITY — STATE ☐☐
97. on campus ○ 1 / off campus ○ 2 / with parent ○ 3

Step Seven: Please read, sign, and date.

By signing this application, you agree, if asked, to provide information that will verify the accuracy of your completed form. This information may include your U.S. or state income tax forms. Also, you certify that you (1) will use federal and/or state student financial aid only to pay the cost of attending an institution of higher education, (2) are not in default on a federal student loan or have made satisfactory arrangements to repay it, (3) do not owe money back on a federal student grant or have made satisfactory arrangements to repay it, (4) will notify your school if you default on a federal student loan, and (5) understand that **the Secretary of Education has the authority to verify information reported on this application with the Internal Revenue Service.** If you purposely give false or misleading information, you may be fined $10,000, sent to prison, or both.

98. Date this form was completed.
MONTH ☐☐ / DAY ☐☐ / 2001 ○ or 2002 ○

99. Student signature (Sign in box)
1 **FOR INFORMATION ONLY.**

Parent signature (one parent whose information is provided in Step Four) (Sign in box)
2 **DO NOT SUBMIT.**

If this form was filled out by someone other than you, your spouse, or your parent(s), that person must complete this part.
Preparer's name, firm, and address
_____
_____
_____

100. Preparer's Social Security Number (or 101)
☐☐☐ — ☐☐ — ☐☐☐☐

101. Employer ID number (or 100)
☐☐ — ☐☐☐☐☐

102. Preparer's signature and date
1

SCHOOL USE ONLY: Federal School Code
D/O ○ 1
FAA SIGNATURE
1 ☐☐☐☐☐☐

MDE USE ONLY:
Special Handle ☐ — ☐☐☐☐☐☐

Notes for questions **59–83** (page 5) **Step Four:** Who is considered a parent in this step?

Read these notes to determine who is considered a parent for purposes of this form. **Answer all questions in Step Four about them,** even if you do not live with them.

If your parents are both living and married to each other, answer the questions about them.

If your parent is widowed or single, answer the questions about that parent. If your widowed parent has remarried as of today, answer the questions about that parent **and** the person whom your parent married (your stepparent).

If your parents have divorced or separated, answer the questions about the parent you lived with more during the past 12 months. (If you did not live with one parent more than the other, give answers about the parent who provided more financial support during the last 12 months, or during the most recent year that you actually received support from a parent.) If this parent has remarried as of today, answer the questions on the rest of this form about that parent **and** the person whom your parent married (your stepparent).

Notes for question **64** (page 5)

Include in your parents' household (see notes, above, for who is considered a parent):
- your parents and yourself, even if you don't live with your parents, and
- your parents' other children if (a) your parents will provide more than half of their support from July 1, 2001 through June 30, 2002 or (b) the children could answer "No" to every question in Step Three, and
- other people if they now live with your parents, your parents provide more than half of their support, and your parents will continue to provide more than half of their support from July 1, 2001 through June 30, 2002.

Notes for questions **65** (page 5) and **85** (page 6)

Always count yourself as a college student. **Do not include your parents.** Include others only if they will attend at least half time in 2001-2002 a program that leads to a college degree or certificate.

Notes for question **84** (page 6)

Include in your (and your spouse's) household:
- yourself (and your spouse, if you have one), and
- your children, if you will provide more than half of their support from July 1, 2001 through June 30, 2002, and
- other people if they now live with you, and you provide more than half of their support, and you will continue to provide more than half of their support from July 1, 2001 through June 30, 2002.

Information on the Privacy Act and use of your Social Security Number

We use the information that you provide on this form to determine if you are eligible to receive federal student financial aid and the amount that you are eligible to receive. Section 483 of the Higher Education Act of 1965, as amended, gives us the authority to ask you and your parents these questions, and to collect the Social Security Numbers of you and your parents.

State and institutional student financial aid programs may also use the information that you provide on this form to determine if you are eligible to receive state and institutional aid and the need that you have for such aid. Therefore, we will disclose the information that you provide on this form to each institution you list in questions 86–97, state agencies in your state of legal residence, and the state agencies of the states in which the colleges that you list in questions 86–97 are located.

If you are applying solely for federal aid, you must answer all of the following questions that apply to you: 1–9, 13–15, 24, 27–28, 31–32, 35, 36–40, 42–49, 52–66, 69–74, 76-85, and 98–99. If you do not answer these questions, you will not receive federal aid.

Without your consent, we may disclose information that you provide to entities under a published "routine use." Under such a routine use, we may disclose information to third parties that we have authorized to assist us in administering the above programs; to other federal agencies under computer matching programs, such as those with the Internal Revenue Service, Social Security Administration, Selective Service System, Immigration and Natural-ization Service, and Veterans Administration; to your parents or spouse; and to members of Congress if you ask them to help you with student aid questions.

If the federal government, the U.S. Department of Education, or an employee of the U.S. Department of Education is involved in litigation, we may send information to the Department of Justice, or a court or adjudicative body, if the disclosure is related to financial aid and certain conditions are met. In addition, we may send your information to a foreign, federal, state, or local enforcement agency if the information that you submitted indicates a violation or potential violation of law, for which that agency has jurisdiction for investigation or prosecution. Finally, we may send information regarding a claim that is determined to be valid and overdue to a consumer reporting agency. This information includes identifiers from the record; the amount, status, and history of the claim; and the program under which the claim arose.

State Certification

By submitting this application, you are giving your state financial aid agency permission to verify any statement on this form and to obtain income tax information for all persons required to report income on this form.

The Paperwork Reduction Act of 1995

The Paperwork Reduction Act of 1995 says that no one is required to respond to a collection of information unless it displays a valid OMB control number, which for this form is 1845-0001. The time required to complete this form is estimated to be one hour, including time to review instructions, search data resources, gather the data needed, and complete and review the information collection. If you have comments about this estimate or suggestions for improving this form, please write to: U.S. Department of Education, Washington DC 20202-4651.

We may request additional information from you to ensure efficient application processing operations. We will collect this additional information only as needed and on a voluntary basis.

Worksheets

Do not mail these worksheets in with your application.
Keep these worksheets; your school may ask to see them.

Worksheet A

Calendar Year 2000

For question 44 Student/Spouse		For question 78 Parent(s)
$	Earned income credit from IRS Form 1040–line 60a; 1040A–line 38a; 1040EZ–line 8a; or Telefile–line L	$
$	Additional child tax credit from IRS Form 1040–line 62 or 1040A–line 39	$
$	Welfare benefits, including Temporary Assistance for Needy Families (TANF). Don't include food stamps.	$
$	Social Security benefits received that were not taxed (such as SSI)	$
$	**Enter in question 44.** **Enter in question 78.**	$

Worksheet B

Calendar Year 2000

For question 45 Student/Spouse		For question 79 Parent(s)
$	Payments to tax-deferred pension and savings plans (paid directly or withheld from earnings), including amounts reported on the W-2 Form in Box 13, codes D, E, F, G, H, and S	$
$	IRA deductions and payments to self-employed SEP, SIMPLE, and Keogh and other qualified plans from IRS Form 1040–total of lines 23 + 29 or 1040A–line 16	$
$	Child support **received** for all children. Don't include foster care or adoption payments.	$
$	Tax exempt interest income from IRS Form 1040–line 8b or 1040A–line 8b	$
$	Foreign income exclusion from IRS Form 2555–line 43 or 2555EZ–line 18	$
$	Untaxed portions of pensions from IRS Form 1040–lines (15a minus 15b) + (16a minus 16b) or 1040A–lines (11a minus 11b) + (12a minus 12b) excluding rollovers	$
$	Credit for federal tax on special fuels from IRS Form 4136–line 9 – nonfarmers only	$
$	Housing, food, and other living allowances paid to members of the military, clergy, and others (including cash payments and cash value of benefits)	$
$	Veterans noneducation benefits such as Disability, Death Pension, or Dependency & Indemnity Compensation (DIC) and/or VA Educational Work-Study allowances	$
$	Any other untaxed income or benefits not reported elsewhere on Worksheets A and B, such as worker's compensation, untaxed portions of railroad retirement benefits, Black Lung Benefits, Refugee Assistance, etc. **Don't include** student aid, Workforce Investment Act educational benefits, or benefits from flexible spending arrangements, e.g., cafeteria plans.	$
$	Cash **received**, or any money paid on your behalf, not reported elsewhere on this form	XXXXXXXX
$	**Enter in question 45.** **Enter in question 79.**	$

Worksheet C

Calendar Year 2000

For question 46 Student/Spouse		For question 80 Parent(s)
$	Education credits (Hope and Lifetime Learning tax credits) from IRS Form 1040-line 46 or 1040A-line 29	$
$	Child support **paid** because of divorce or separation. Do not include support for children in your (or your parents') household, as reported in question 84 (or question 64 for your parents).	$
$	Taxable earnings from Federal Work-Study or other need-based work programs	$
$	Student grant, scholarship, and fellowship aid, including AmeriCorps awards, that was reported to the IRS in your (or your parents') adjusted gross income	$
$	**Enter in question 46.** **Enter in question 80.**	$

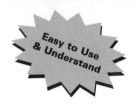
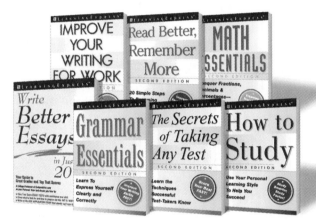
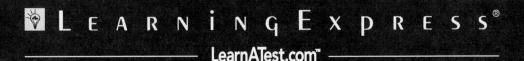